ACKNOWLEGEMENTS

Many people have contributed ideas and techniques during the years of my clinical work leading to development of the concepts in this book. I wish to thank Linda West RN, Gail Nevin PT, Catherine Goodman, PT, Anna Furshong PT, Barbara Penner PT, and Gayle Cochran Phram.D. who have consistently provided support and stimulation for my ideas. I appreciate the ideas therapists have provided while participating in my courses on pelvic pain, especially Diane Olhoeft PT, Kathleen Vosburgh PT, Tammy Fegely, Margaret Moffatt PT, Betsy Hart, OTR/L, Maribeth Johnson PT, Mary Thane PT, Sidney Whitsell PT, and Amber Coulter PT. My patients through the years have taught me which ideas work and those to never mention again. You are the best editor of self care in existence. Last, but not least, I thank my family John, Richard, Erika and Abigail for their expert advise about real people and their bravery and fortitude in working with pain and disability.

Other publications
by the author

Fibromyalgia
A Handbook for Self Care & Treatment
3rd Edition

Beyond Kegels
Fabulous four exercises and more...
to prevent and treat incontinence

Beyond Kegels Book II
Treatment Algorithms
&
Special Populations

Geriatric Incontinence
A Behavioral and Exercise Approach
to Treatment

Table of Contents

INTRODUCTION

Chronic pelvic pain with low back pain is a significant diagnosis in women from adolescence through adulthood. The chronic pain may be constant or recurrent but in either instance it alters social, personal and working relationships as well as requiring limitless medical attention for a condition that often seems unsolvable. The diagnosis of chronic pelvic pain with low back pain needs to be considered a disease entity in itself rather than a group of sub-diagnoses with similar symptoms. This allows for the assessment and treatment paradigms to focus on self-care and management rather than the assessment and treatment paradigms focusing on a cure for a specific condition.

This book is developed with the acknowledgement of self-care and management as an underlying foundation for effective medical intervention. The first section of the book delineates the conditions, definitions, symptoms and possible triggers of chronic pelvic pain with low back pain. The second section describes the anatomy, physiology and neurology that can be involved in chronic pelvic pain. The third section develops effective assessment techniques that include history and special questions, and physical assessment with special tests and considerations. Finally, section four describes basic and advanced self-care management as well as medical intervention strategies for effective treatment of chronic pelvic pain with low back pain.

The first and second sections develop background information and rationale for the assessment and treatment sections that follow. The third section is designed for the medical professional to use in determining priority areas during treatment. It includes sequential outlines and forms for a comprehensive assessment that directs self-care management. The fourth section provides a step-by-step approach to basic self-care using self-monitoring tests and progessive self-stabilizing loops of care. Once the basic self-care stabilizing loop becomes part of daily life, the advanced techniques can be beneficial in taking the individual to the next level of independence from pain, fatigue and isolation.

This book is written for both the health care professional and the individual with chronic pelvic pain. Sections one, two and four can be of interest to both individuals. Section three is primarily oriented to the health care professional. The words may be technical but the self-care concepts are practical and realistic for individuals with chronic pelvic pain. Hundreds of patients have seen their lives improve with these protocols. When chronic pelvic pain with low back pain is conceptualized as a valuable part of the individual and self-care and treatment is based on physiological principles, the improvement seen can be impressive and life altering.

Chapter 1

Description, Criteria and Symptoms

Description

Chronic pelvic pain (CPP) is defined as persistent pain of unexplained nature in the lower abdominal and pelvic area. It is pelvic pain without evidence of active disease or pathology that is six months or longer in duration and effects physical activity, work, family and social life in a negative way.

Criteria

The criteria are:

Duration	• lasting 6 months or longer
Etiology	• lacks apparent physical cause to explain pain
	• tests are not indicative of cause
Functional	• decreased physical function and
Level	interaction with the environment

Pain Characteristics and Location

Individuals describe a variety of pain levels and types. Pain varies between 5 and 10 on a 0 to 10 scale. Pain levels 5 and above effect physical activity, work, family and social life in a negative way. Chronic pelvic pain can be located in the pelvis, genital, rectal, abdominal, coccyx, sacral and/or low back areas. Pain can be referred to the low back and lower extremities.

Types of Pain

There are 3 types of pelvic pain including somatic, visceral and neuropathic pain.

Somatic pain is the most familiar to individuals. It is pain coming from the skin and transmitted to the brain in the cerebral cortex where it is perceived as very localized and sharp or stinging pain. The response of the body part is to withdraw from the pain stimulus. If the pain is in the abdomen, the abdominal muscles tighten. If the pain is in the pelvis the pelvic muscles tighten. For the most part the pain is perceived objectively not emotionally.

Visceral pain comes from the internal organs including the bladder, bowel, uterus and parietal peritoneum. It is due to stretching, distension, or inflammation of tissues with nerve innervation within the abdominal cavity. Visceral pain is transmitted through the spinal cord to the central portion of the brain called the limbic system. It is perceived by the individual as emotional- dreadful, excruciating, or just plain terrible. Visceral pain leads to withdrawal and avoidance behaviors. Individuals experience decreased social interaction and work activity levels as well as depression, as directed by the limbic system.

Neuropathic pain comes from specific nerve fibers that are effected in some way. It can be due to compression, stretching, tearing or cutting, or interruption of blood supply to the nerve. It is often associated with a loss of sensation in the area experiencing pain. Neuropathic pain is described as having a burning or electrical quality. The pain can be stimulated by light touch or vibration. The pain travels to brain centers and results in emotional symptoms as well as physical withdrawal.

Associated Problems

Chronic pelvic pain is often associated with low back pain, constipation and/or voiding dysfunctions such as a small stream flow, urgency, frequency, or difficulty starting or stopping urine. The pain is often exacerbated by sitting. In females, dyspareunia (painful intercourse) and sexual dysfunction (lack of orgasm) are associated with CPP.

Low Back Pain and Chronic Pelvic Pain

Low back pain (LBP) is commonly seen in association with CPP. Low back pain can be caused by stenosis, disc degeneration, joint dysfunction, muscle spasm, nerve compression or ischemia. It can also be a referred pain from visceral pathology or dysfunction. Even though LBP is an associated symptom in many subcategories of CPP, lumbosacral pathology is rarely the cause of CPP except during pregnancy according to Howard.

Lumbo-pelvic dysfunction is often the result of instability in the region. Alteration in function of the passive, active or control segments of the lumbo-pelvic region can result in pain, movement disorders, and postural changes. The dynamic stabilization of the lumbo-sacral region by integrated muscle action enables effective movement and weight transmittal through the neutral zone of stabilized joint structures. According to Lee the pelvis becomes the fulcrum from which lever arms of the lower extremities and spine move. This book describes the interaction of the pelvic muscle force field (PMFF) with other active segments during movement in the lumbo-pelvic region. In most major functional activities, whether it is standing, walking, bending, or reaching, the lumbo-pelvic dynamic stability is dependent on the pelvic muscle force field. In dysfunction, the lumbo-pelvic region in conjunction with the pelvic muscle force field contributes to CPP and limitation of daily activities.

Chapter 2

Diagnostic Categories

Chronic pelvic pain, by definition, does not have a definite cause identified by a specific test or surgery. There are physical and psychological factors that contribute to and perpetuate CPP.

Physical factors can include:

Endometriosis, pelvic adhesions, pelvic inflammatory disease, pelvic varicosities, pelvic congestion, organ malposition, nerve entrapment or damage, musculoskeletal dysfunction, myofascial dysfunction (myofascial pain syndrome), cystitis, or fibromyalgia.

Psychological factors can include:

Psychosomatic disorders, depression, sexual abuse, sexual dysfunction, personality disorder, or neurosis.

How Is It Diagnosed? Who Has It?

How Is It Diagnosed?

Chronic pelvic pain is diagnosed through a history, a pain diagram, and negative medical test results. Tests for tumors, cancer, inflammation, infection, and neurological deficits are inconclusive or negative in CPP.

Who has it?

One in every seven women between the age of 18 and 50 has experienced pelvic pain. Chronic pelvic pain effects more women than men.

What Are The Diagnoses?

Chronic pelvic pain syndromes can be divided into pelvic muscle myalgia (pain) syndromes, pelvic muscle relaxation syndromes, urological (bladder) syndromes, and other syndromes.

Pelvic Muscle Myalgia Syndromes

Pelvic Muscle Myalgia Syndromes include:
  Levator Ani Syndrome
  Piriformis Syndrome
  Coccygodynia
  Vaginisimus
  Dyspareunia
  Proctalgia Fugax
  Vulvodynia
  Vulvar Vestibulitis Syndrome
  Pudendal Neuralgia

Pelvic Muscle Myalgia Syndrome is sometimes termed pelvic myalgia. In general it includes increased resting tone of levator ani, coccygeus, medial fibers of gluteus, piriformis and/or obturator internus. There is pain around the rectum, in the low back, vagina, coccyx, and posterior thigh.

Causes can include genitourinary inflammation, rectal dysfunctions or diseases such as fissures and hemorrhoids, post surgical sequelae from laminectomy or hysterectomy, pelvic fracture, trauma to sacrum or coccyx, or head trauma.

Levator Ani Syndrome is described by individuals as pain and pressure in the rectal and vaginal areas. There is often unilateral pain on the left side more than the right. Defecation can promote pain and throbbing in the rectal and vaginal areas. There is increased resting tone of the levator ani (pelvic diaphragm) muscle group. The resting tone does not relax or release appropriately when the individual attempts to have a bowel movement or urinate. The result can be difficulty initiating urination and defecation and straining to have a bowel movement.

Causes include previous pelvic surgery, strenuous physical activity, injury during childbirth, lumbar disc surgery, pelvic infection or inflammation, or sexual assault injury.

Piriformis Syndrome is described by individuals as pain in the buttocks extending into the rectal area. Pain is often referred into the posterior aspect of the thigh and sometimes into the calf musculature.

Coccygodynia is described by individuals as pain around the tailbone region (coccyx). There can be referred pain into the posterior buttocks and the posterior thigh. There is often difficulty sitting for any length of time.

Causes can include a coccyx injury from a fall or during childbirth or surgery, arthritic changes in joint structures, spasm of coccygeus muscle or pirformis muscle, or neuralgia or neuritis of the coccygeal nerve plexus.

Vaginisimus is described by individuals as pain and spasm around the vaginal opening when there is an attempt to penetrate the vagina. There is increased tone of the superficial muscles (urogenital diaphragm muscles) and the deeper muscles (levator ani/pelvic diaphragm muscles). There is recurrent or persistent involuntary spasm of the musculature around the outer one third of the vagina that interferes with coitus and sexual function.

Causes can include physical and psychological factors. It can be a protective response to atrophic vaginitis (hypoestrogenation). The vaginal walls thin and lose lubrication due to the decreased estrogen levels of perimenopause and menopause. Any penetration causes abrasions and irritation when there is inadequate estrogen available to the tissues. This occurs most often in women after 45-50 years of age. Vaginisimus can also be a protective response to a hole in the wall of the vagina, called a fistula. Psychological factors include a response to past sexual abuse, physical abuse or other trauma.

Dyspareunia is described by individuals as pain localized to the vagina and lower pelvis before, during, or immediately after intercourse. Symptoms are caused by initial penetration or deep penetration. The pain can be intermittent or persistent. Dyspareunia can prevent intercourse and use of tampons.

Causes of dyspareunia can include physical and psychological factors. Physical causes include nerve damage, physical and sexual trauma to pelvic muscles. Psychological aspects that cause dyspareunia include past sexual abuse, physical abuse or other trauma.

Proctalgia fugax is described by individuals as sharp fleeting rectal pain lasting from 20-30 seconds to several hours. There can be an accumulation of flatus in the rectum. These symptoms occur more at night, during straining with bowel movements and during or after intercourse. There is spasm of the levator ani, specifically the puborectalis muscle and external anal sphincter. There can be a circulatory disturbance in the surrounding anal muscles. Proctalgia fugax affects men more than women. There is no known cause for proctalgia fugax.

Vulvodynia and vulvar vestibulitis syndromes are described by individuals as burning, stinging irritation, and/or rawness in the vaginal and labia area. The discomfort is unremitting and consuming. The skin around the opening of the vagina often appears normal or only slightly red. The symptoms can prevent the individual from wearing clothing, walking, or participating in intercourse due to the hypersensitivity in the perineal area. There is extreme pain with touch or pressure around the labia and vaginal opening. The symptoms rarely awaken the individual at night. There is no definite cause for vulvodynia.

Pudendal neuralgia is described by individuals as nearly constant burning pain in the saddle region (through the perineum and a line connecting the ischial tuberosities, extending into the lateral upper thighs). Light touch can provoke intense symptoms which include itching, numbness, and a sensation of dryness in the clitoris, urethral opening, vulva and labia, the perineum, and rectal region. There are no skin changes.

The cause is irritation of the internal pudendal nerve which provides sensation to the perineal area, lateral upper thighs, and rectal area. The causative factors include pressure, ischemia or damage to the nerve during surgery or vaginal delivery, trauma, or extreme edema.

Pelvic Muscle Relaxation Syndromes

Pelvic Muscle Relaxation Syndromes include:
Cystocele
Urethrocele
Enterocele
Recotocele
Vaginal Prolapse
Uterine Prolapse

Pelvic Muscle Relaxation Syndromes are described by individuals as pelvic and back pain in general. More specifically a painful, heavy, downward dragging feeling is experienced in the groin and pelvis as well as sacral backache from uterosacral ligament traction on the sacrum.

Cystocele is the collapse of the bladder which descends down the vaginal canal. In addition to the general pelvic muscle relaxation syndrome symptoms, individuals with cystocele can experience leaking, frequency, and urgency. Persistent urinary tract infections are common.

Urethrocele is the collapse of the urethra which descends down the vaginal canal.

Enterocele is the collapse of the intestines which descends down the vaginal canal.

Rectocele is the collapse of the rectum which descends down the vaginal canal. An individual with rectocele describes difficulty emptying the rectum. As the individual bears down to push the stool out it instead is pushed into the rectocele. The harder the individual pushes the larger the rectocele becomes. Constipation is another common symptom.

Vaginal prolapse is the collapse of the vagina toward or through the vaginal opening after a hysterectomy.

Uterine prolapse is the descent of the uterus toward or through the vaginal opening.

Retroversion of the uterus is the posterior displacement of the uterus and rarely results in pain in and of itself. The pain described is primarily due to dyspareunia and low back, sacral pain.

Urological Syndromes

Urological Syndromes include:
Urethral Syndrome
Trigonitis
Bladder-Sphincter Dysenergia
Interstitial Cystitis
Prostatitis

Urological Syndromes involve pain and dysfunction of smooth muscles of the bladder and urethra in conjunction with hypertonus of the pelvic muscles. The most troublesome symptoms besides pain include urgency, frequency, nocturia (night-time wetting), pressure, voiding difficulty, dysuria (abnormal urine flow), constipation, and fatigue.

Urethral Syndrome is described by individuals as pain, burning and hypersensitivity around the urethra. This is accompanied by urinary frequency, urgency and hesitancy. Frequency is the primary complaint with a constant awareness of the urethra. Toileting is slow and hesitant. Nocturia (night-time leaking) is mild to absent. There may be narrowing of the urethral tube by muscles or fascia. Sexual activity can cause irritation as can hypoestrogenation. Pelvic fractures and complications post bladder suspension surgery have been factors in urethral syndrome.

Trigonitis is described by individuals as discomfort and urgency sensation with pressure on the lower bladder. This often occurs during intercourse if there is urine retention and with atrophic changes from hypoestrogenation.

Bladder-Sphincter Dysenergia is described by individuals as the urge to toilet yet when on the toilet the urine flow is not present or difficult to initiate. The bladder contracts simultaneously with the outlet contracting.

Interstitial Cystitis (IC) is described by individuals as suprapubic (lower abdominal) pressure and pain accompanied by urgency and frequency. Individuals with interstitial cystitis often toilet every 30 minutes during the day and more than three times at night. They describe being limited in daily activities due to frequent toileting and sleep deprivation.

There is no known etiology or pathogenesis. There is an absence of other pathology along with the voiding symptoms and characteristic bladder lining changes. The median age of onset is 40 but 25% of individuals with IC experience symptoms before 30.

Prostatitis is described by individuals as suprapubic (lower abdominal) and gonad pain and discomfort that is accompanied by urgency and frequency. When at the toilet the urine flow is not present or is difficult to start. Pain is severe enough that sitting for any period of time is difficult. Acute prostatitis is a bacterial infection and requires treatment with antibiotics. Chronic benign prostatitis exhibits the symptomotology without the bacterial infection.

Chapter 3

Triggers For Chronic Pelvic Pain and Low Back Pain

Possible triggers for CPP can include:
Visceral Organ Dysfunction
Pelvic Congestion Syndrome/Pelvic Varicosities
Neurally Mediated Hypotension
Reproductive Hormone Imbalance
Peripheral Myofascial Trigger Points
Skeletal Joint Dysfunction
Fibromyalgia Hernias
Nerve Entrapment/Neuropathy
Post Hysterectomy Chronic Pain
Post Traumatic Stress Disorder
Fibroid Tumors
Hypoglycemia Tendencies
Hypothyroid Tendencies

Visceral Organ Dysfunction is described by individuals as deep nonspecific pain within the pelvis as well as referred pain to the lower abdomen and low back bilaterally. The dysfunction or pathology can be from the bladder, uterus, bowel, rectum, anus, or connective tissues such as fascia, ligament, blood vessels, nerve, and parietal peritoneum.

Pelvic Congestion Syndrome/Pelvic Varicosities is described by individuals as dull, aching pelvic pain similar to that produced by varicosities in the legs. The pain is intermittent, brought on by simple activities. It is most often dull, aching, unilateral and located in the lateral lower abdominal and low back area. It is most severe premenstrually. Low back pain in the sacral area is often made worse by standing and improved by reclining. Menstrual pain and pain during intercourse often accompany this syndrome. Nausea, flatulence and gastric distress have been described. Bladder symptoms include frequency, urgency and burning with urination. Headache, fatigue, and insomnia have also been described. This syndrome is characterized by dilated, incompetent ovarian veins that accumulate blood causing stasis due to incompetent valves. Premenstrual hormone changes, pregnancy, and genetic predisposition can cause the varicosities.

Neurally Mediated Hypotension (NMH) is described by individuals as abdominal pain that mimics the pain from gall stones, interstitial cystitis, endometriosis, or cancer so well that abdominal surgery is performed. The individual experiences extreme abdominal pain, low blood pressure and high resting heart rate. Fatigue, dizziness, feeling weak in the knees and unsteady when rising from a reclined position or sitting are characteristics of NMH. This syndrome is closely related to Pelvic Congestion/Pelvic Varicosities in that the hypotension can lead to pooling of blood in the pelvic veins with the resultant symptoms.

Reproductive Hormone Imbalance is described by individuals as monthly and/or yearly cycles of incapacitating abdominal pain, fatigue, sleep disturbance, menstrual irregularities, bowel and bladder irritability and depression. The symptoms are experienced in the week prior to menstruation on a monthly cycle and often exhibit increased severity in the transition time between fall and winter or winter and spring. Estrogen and progesterone levels vary on a monthly cycle and a yearly cycle. They gradually rise during the first half of the monthly cycle, fall at mid cycle (day fourteen), and rise again the last half of the 28-day-cycle until falling as a stimulus for menstruation. Yearly variations in estrogen and progesterone include elevations in spring going into summer and decline during fall going into winter.

Peripheral Myofascial Trigger Points are described by individuals as lower abdominal, pelvic and low back pain. It can be intermittent pain brought on by physical activity. Muscles with trigger points that can refer pain into the pelvic region include those in the abdomen, low back, buttocks, anterior, medial and posterior thighs.

Muscles and symptoms include:

Obliques–heartburn, projectile vomiting, diarrhea, and belching, lower quadrant and groin pain.

Rectus Abdominus–bilateral horizontal midback and upper buttock pain, lower right quadrant pain in the region of McBurney's point, dysmenorrhea, abdominal fullness, nausea, and vomiting.

Pectineus–deep groin pain especially with weight bearing and abduction.

Adductors–deep groin pain, internal pelvic pain and pain into the anterior medial thigh.

Quadratus Lumborum–low back pain from the 12th rib to the iliac crest, sacroiliac joint into the buttock; lower abdominal and groin area are secondary pain areas.

Iliopsoas–ipsilateral back pain from 12th rib to sacroiliac joint, lower abdomen, groin, anterior superior thigh.

Obturator Internus–internal pelvic pain in the vagina and rectum, pain around the coccyx, anal sphincter, and extending down the ipsilateral posterior thigh.

Levator Ani–pain around the coccyx and anal sphincter.

Anal and Vaginal Sphincters- poorly localized pain in the anal region, painful bowel movements, entry dyspareunia, vaginisimus.

Gluteus Maximus–pain in the buttocks, lower sacrum amd coccyx into the ischial tuberosity area.

Piriformis–pain in sacral coccyx area extending to lateral buttock and posterior thigh.

Skeletal Joint Dysfunction is described by individuals as pain in the abdomen, low back, and pelvic region that increases with movement, standing and sitting. The symptoms can extend into the anterior, medial or posterior thigh.

Joints that may be involved include:

Symphysis Pubis–pain over the pubic rami, lower abdomen, groin and deep pelvic region.

Sacroiliac–pain in the deep pelvic region, sacral and buttock areas.

Lumbar facets–pain in lower abdomen and buttocks extending to posterior thigh.

Fibromyalgia is described by individuals as lower abdominal, pelvic and low back pain acommpanied by sleep disturbance, fatigue, urinary frequency, urgency and leaking.

Hernias are described by individuals as a bulge and pressure with pain and dragging feeling in the area of the hernia. There are three types of hernias. Abdominal wall hernias - epgastric, umbilical, Spigelian and incisional hernias. Groin hernias- inguinal and femoral hernias. Pelvic wall and pelvic floor hernias- sciatic, obturator, and perineal hernias. Those that can lead to pelvic pain include sciatic, obturator, perineal, inguinal, epigastric(linea alba), umbilical, Spigelian, and incisional. The sciatic hernia is described as one sided pelvic pain that can extend into the buttock and posterior thigh. Obturator hernias results in pelvic pain and pain down the inner thigh into the knee joint and at times the hip joint. Perineal hernia is rarely accompanied by severe pain, rather some individuals describe minor discomfort with urination or discomfort while sitting. Inguinal hernias can predispose an individual to minor, even severe pain as well as a sickening feeling in the pit of the stomach. Femoral hernias are rarely the cause of pelvic pain. Hernias of the linea alba (epigastric hernias) can cause colicky pain, nausea, and vomiting. Umbilical hernias can lead to severe pain with coughing or straining. Spigelian hernias, within the abdominal muscle and fascial layers, can precipitate sharp constant or intermittent pain and a dragging feeling. Incisional hernias can lead to nausea, vomiting, and intermittent pain. Internal pelvic hernias can lead to general abdominal pain, bloating and tenderness.

Nerve Entrapment/Neuropathy is described by individuals as constant, burning pain, sensory loss, tingling or hypersensitivity in specific areas of the abdomen, pelvis, or thigh. Iliohypogastric and ilioinguinal neuropathies are experienced most often immediately after surgery. Pain is described as burning or shooting throughout the lower abdomen radiating to the labia or inner thigh. Tenderness is often present medial to the anterior superior iliac spine (the point of entrapment). Hypersensitivity is more common than numbness. Genitofemoral neuropathy is described as pain, hypersensitivity, and numbness in the medial inguinal area extending to the inner thigh and labia. Lateral femoral cutaneous neuropathy is described as pain in the lower abdomen, groin and anterolateral thigh. In all of the above conditions standing, walking, and bending can increase pain.

Pudendal neuralgia varies from vague to well defined pain in the perineum, groin and leg. Hypersensitivity to light touch can be extreme. External anal sphincter dysfunction can lead to fecal incontinence. The pudendal nerve is affected during the second stage of labor (delivery), cycling, and horseback riding. Obturator neuropathy is described as pain and/or numbness along the medial thigh. It can occur with compression of the fetal head during a difficult delivery. Femoral neuropathy is described as pain and/or numbness in the area of the anterior thigh. Sciatic neuropathy is described as pain down the posterior leg and at times into the pelvic region.

The cause of neuropathies in the abdominal-pelvic region can be pressure, stretch, direct trauma or entrapment. The nerve may be compressed as it passes through a canal or notch or as it travels between tight fascial bands or through muscle fiber bundles. The result is nerve ischemia (lack of oxygen to the nerve) as its vascular supply is decreased or obliterated. Demyelinization can also occur with pressure of a more severe nature. Stretch injury occurs most often during labor and delivery but also occurs during abdominal or pelvic surgery when a rupture of some nerve fibers cause an extreme stretch. After nerve damage there can be regeneration of nerve endings- called sprouting. These sprouts become extremely sensitive to any stimuli.

Post Hysterectomy Chronic Pain is often described by an individual as sharp, stinging, burning or tingling pain during intercourse or certain physical activities. It may be cyclical in nature following the menstrual cycle. When hysterectomy is performed to relieve pelvic pain it is effective 75% of the time. Despite these positive results there are women who after hysterectomy have chronic pain. Post hysterectomy pain can occur from the vaginal apex, a residual or remnant ovary, adhesions, or remnant endometriosis. When there is a problem with the vagina at the distal surgical site it is called deep dyspareunia (pain with intercourse) and is described as sharp, stinging, burning, or tingling. The origin of the pain can be from lack of adequate vaginal expansion due to decreased sexual arousal, an inclusional cyst, chronic stitch abscess, or remnant endometriosis in the vaginal cuff. Pain from a residual ovary is often due to cyst formation in the ovary. This pain is most often cyclical following the hormonal changes of the menstrual cycle. Even when the ovary is removed, there may be a remnant inadvertently left that can exhibit itself as pelvic pain. Postoperative adhesions are present after hysterectomy but they do not always cause pain. The pain from adhesions can be from the pull of the adhesions on the parietal peritoneum or from the adhesions themselves that have developed their own vascular supply. Endometriosis is a common diagnosis that results in hysterectomy. Approximately 10% of these women experience a recurrence of symptoms. This may be due to recurrent endometriosis or any of the other mechanisms previously mentioned.

Post Traumatic Stress Disorder pain is described by individuals as a wide variety of pain types and dysfunctions in the abdominal, pelvic and low back region. Bladder and bowel function is often effected. Sleep disturbance, hypervigilence, and a feeling of "disease" are described. The symptoms may result from autonomic nervous system response to sexual and/or physical abuse during childhood or adulthood, muscle holding patterns, or injury to soft tissues in the pelvic region.

Fibroid Tumors (leiomyomas) pain is described by individuals as a feeling of pressure, urinary frequency or leaking, cramping uterine pain, or intermittent pain from the parietal perineum. There is often heavy menstruation significant enough to bleed through any protection. Fibroid tumors are the most common tumors found in women. These tumors are present within the uterus. Rapid growth or degeneration of these tumors occur with the hormonal changes of pregnancy and menopause. Generally these tumors are asymptomatic but symptoms can occur if blood supply is compromised or if they pull on other innervated tissue.

Hypoglycemia or **Reactive Hypoglycemia Tendencies** is described by individuals as feeling shaky, dizzy, irritable, irrational and weak. Other symptoms include headache, pelvic and abdominal pain, depression, anxiety, sweet cravings, confusion, night sweats, and insomnia. These individuals can become aggressive and easily lose their tempers during a hypoglycemic episode. Stress increases metabolism, activating insulin and glucose release.

Hypothyroid Tendencies are described by individuals as feeling cold (cold hands and feet, feeling core cold), weight gain, dry skin, heavy menstruation, PMS, and constipation. Additional complaints include fatigue, sleep disturbance, and pelvic and abdominal pain. These descriptors may be caused by hypothyroid tendencies, a sluggish thyroid gland that is not producing adequate thyroid hormone or dysfunction of thyroid hormone at the cellular level. Thyroid hormone produced by the thyroid gland is an essential information molecule for many body functions. Another essential thyroid hormone is produced primarily at the cellular tissue level from hormones originating from the thyroid gland.

Chapter 4

Causative Factors and Physiology

Research has discovered that individuals with CPP can have alterations in several of the chemical messengers in their blood stream, spinal fluid, and urine as compared to normal individuals. Most of these chemical assays are primarily performed in research labs and are not available in clinical situations. Research has also discovered that specific body systems are functioning abnormally in CPP. These systems include the:

- hypothalamic-pituitary-adrenal axis
- autonomic nervous system axis, and
- reproductive hormone axis

Necklaces as Chemical Messengers

Chemical messengers maintain brain activity, they regulate mood, control sleep, appetite, memory, and mental alterness. Chemical messengers regulate muscle action, gut action, breathing patterns and heart rate. Chemical messengers determine energy levels, metabolic rate, and pain levels.

Most of the chemical messengers are formed from molecules of amino acids which come from proteins.

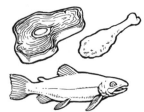

When protein is eaten it is digested and broken into 20-30 different amino acids. (Figure 1)

These different amino acids combine into chains similar to necklaces. There are many combinations of amino acid chains just like there are many different kinds of necklaces. These chains of amino acids are called polypeptides. Familiar polypeptides include serotonin, enkephalins and insulin.

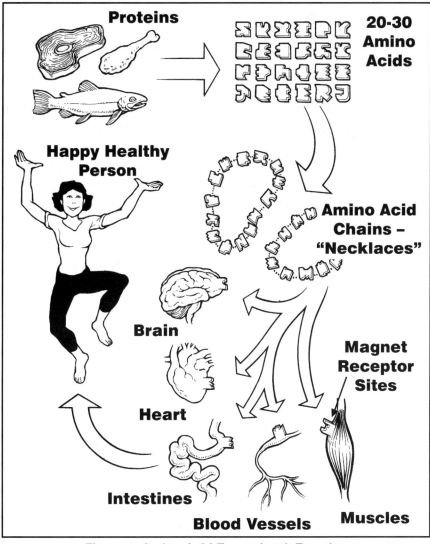

Figure 1: Amino Acid Formation & Function

Manufacturing, Transporting, Receiving of Necklaces

The chemical messengers – amino acid chains – are manufactured at many sites throughout the body. They are manufactured in the brain, in glands like the thyroid, in organs like the pancreas and liver, in the digestive system, in the heart and ciruclatory system and in the muscles. A certain amino acid chain may be manufactured primarily at one site but will also have several other minor manufacturing "plants" at other sites. For example, 95% of serotonin is produced in the gut but there are also manufacturing sites for serotonin in the brain and the muscles. Insulin is produced primarily in the pancreas but also in the brain and muscles.

These chemical messengers are transported via the blood stream or nerve fibers to many different receptor-magnet-sites where they regulate body functions. When they are present in nerve fibers they are known as neurotransmitters, in the blood stream they are known as hormones or biochemicals. Receptor-magnet-sites for specific amino acid chains may be primarily on one organ or in one system but there will be multiple sites throughout the body with minor receptor-magnet-sites. For example, receptor-magnet-sites for serotonin are found in the pancreas, the intestines, the brain, and the heart.

What Can Go Wrong with Necklaces?

The amino acid chains attached to receptor-magnet-sites activate and regulate organs and body systems that allow the human body and mind to function efficiently and without pain or fatigue. What can happen to alter this process?

- There may not be enough amino acid chains due to inadequate "raw materials" or precursors, i.e. proteins, vitamins, and minerals.
- There may be an inefficient manufacturing of protein to amino acid chains leading to excessive need for more and more proteins and amino acids.
- There may be an excessive destruction of the chemical

messengers before they have delivered the essential messages to the receptor-magnet-sites.

- There may be excessive production of the chemical messengers so they drown the receiving sites instead of providing important information on a gradual basis.
- The receptor sites may not be properly sensitive. The receptor-magnet-sites may not be powerful enough to attract and use the chemical messengers that arrive at the site.

Any disruption in the manufacturing, distribution, or use of these messengers results in body and mind dysfunction – pain, fatigue, memory problems, sleep disruption, sensory hypersensitivity, blood pressure changes, or digestive changes.

What Environmental Triggers Can Break the Necklaces?

Environmental triggers can set off CPP and are often described as "causing" CPP. A motor vehicle accident, repetitive motion injury at work, divorce, birth or death, surgery, sexual abuse or infection can act as the trigger that sets off the cascade of symptoms based on the underlying problem of the chemical messaging system. Previously the body had been accommodating for the CPP, keeping the symptoms to a minimum, maintaining the balance within body functions until the trigger "upset the applecart" as the saying goes. Once the trigger sets off the waterfall of symptoms it is difficult to reverse the process unless the underlying problem is understood.

Genetics and the Environment to Produce the Best Necklaces

We are ultimately products of both our genetics and our environment. What happens in our lives triggers or inhibits genetic tendencies. If our genes predispose us to pain and fatigue we must minimize these tendencies through environmental interventions. This is no different than if genetics predispose an individual to be overweight. To minimize the genetic tendency for being overweight, increased exercise and decreased food intake is a necessity. In CPP the genetic tendency for disruption in the manufacturing, distribution, and/or use of amino acid messenger chains can be greatly exacerbated by environmental triggers. For CPP individuals to experienece minimal symptoms requires environmental modification – life style changes – to minimize the disruption in the messaging system.

Whose Job Is This Anyway?

The human body is regulated by control centers using the amino acid necklaces or fatty acid necklaces as chemical messengers. A disturbance in any one of these centers affects the other systems and the functioning of the human as a whole. Disturbances in three of these control systems have been identified in CPP individuals. The three systems are:

The Hypothalamic - Pituitary - Adrenal Axis (HPA)
The Autonomic Nervous System Axis (ANS)
The Reproductive Hormone Axis (RHA)

These three systems function independently to some extent but also influence each other on a regular basis. (Figure 2) Each system provides information and regulation to every cell in the body. Each system provides regulatory influence to the other two systems. Dysfunction in one system can influence dysfunction in the other two systems as well as disrupting general body cellular function.

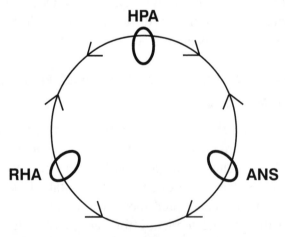

Figure 2: Interaction of HPA, ANS & RHA Axis

Hypothalamic - Pituitary - Adrenal (HPA) Axis

The Stress Axis

The hypothalamic - pituitary-adrenal axis is considered the stress system of the body because the chemical messengers given off by this combination of glands

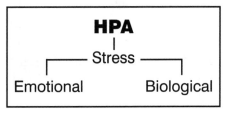

effect the body's ability to cope with stress, both emotional and biological. (Figure 3) Biological stress includes dysfunction in metabolic and physiologic processes controlling blood pressure, blood sugar, and infection control. The hypothalamus, pituitary and adrenal glands produce chemical messengers that modulate pain, sleep, mood, sex drive, appetite, energy, and circulation.

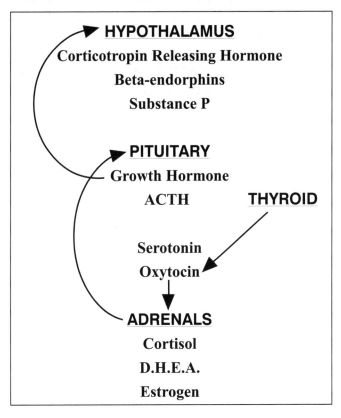

Figure 3: HPA Axis Hormones

Many of the HPA axis hormones are found to be at abnormal levels in CPP. The individuals' cerebral spinal fluid is found to have serotonin in decreased amounts and Substance P is found in increased amounts. Growth hormone and cortisol are also found to be lower than normal in CPP. Dysfunction within the HPA axis can lead to CPP symptoms. When these chemical messengers are at abnormal levels the CPP individual experiences pain, sleep, mood, and energy changes.

The Autonomic Nervous System (ANS)

ANS

Sympathetic Nervous System	Enteric Nervous System	Parasympathetic Nervous System

The autonomic nervous system is the control system sending messages from the brain to organs like the heart, lungs, intestines, bowel, and bladder. There are three subdivisions of the autonomic nervous system: the sympathetic, the parasympathetic and the enteric divisions. These are named for the locations from which they come. The sympathetic system comes from the thoracic and lumbar areas of the spine, the parasympathetic system comes from the cranial and sacral areas of the spine, and the enteric originates from the digestive system or gut. Contrary to popular belief, the sympathetic system is not always defined as excitatory, fight or flight, and the parasympathetic is not always quieting in nature. The parasympathetic nervous system is faster and more localized in its influence on the body. The sympathetic nervous system is slower and more widespread in its influence on the body systems. The parasympathetic nervous system action is more often restricted to a single organ while the sympathetic nervous system action more often effects the body as a whole. The enteric nervous system regulates intestinal or gut function and is the least known and understood division of the autonomic nervous system.

The autonomic nervous system (ANS) and the HPA axis work together effecting each other and all other body systems. Norepinephrine (adrenaline) and neuropeptide Y produced in the ANS facilitate action in the HPA axis. Together the ANS and HPA axes influence areas of the brain involved in cognitive function, memory, memory retrieval and emotional analysis of experiences.

The Sympathetic and Parasympathetic Divisions

The heart, lungs, stomach, liver, pancreas, bladder, uterus, rectum and anus are all directed by sympathetic and parasympathetic divisions of the autonomic nervous system. When there is pain and dysfunction related to these organs, the autonomic nervous system will be involved in either a direct or indirect way. There is most often an imbalance between the parasympathetic and sympathetic input to organ function. Excitatory, survival messages of the sympathetic system to organs become more predominant and enduring rather than a balance of excitatory and quieting directions that allow the organs to work and rest in a healthy rhythm. This imbalance in ANS messaging and the resultant organ response leads initially to super efficient organ function at high energy levels. But as with any machine or body system, rest and maintenance is essential, and in this picture there is little or no rest/maintenance cycle. The result is an eventual melt down of organ function with the symptoms described by the individual as pain, fatigue, indigestion, diarrhea, shortness of breath and menstrual irregularity.

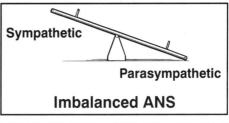

The muscles of the arms, legs, back and trunk are also influenced by the ANS. At rest these voluntary muscles have some tone/tension. The amount or degree of tone/tension present when the muscles are at rest is determined to a large

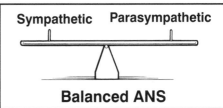

extent by the sympathetic portion of the ANS. The muscle spindle functions much like a spring. The spring can be set tight or loose. If the spring is set tight the muscle has high resting tone. If the spring is set loose the muscle has low resting tone. The ANS sets the tightness or looseness of the spring. When the ANS is dysfunctional it will influence the muscles resulting in abnormally high resting tone. This effects the ability of muscles to work and rest efficiently and effectively.

Returning a balance to the sympathetic-parasympathetic divisions of the ANS is essential in improving CPP symptoms.

The Enteric Division

An Electrical Messaging System From The Gut

The enteric division of the ANS is the gut's control system, or the "gut brain," and lines the digestive system from the esophagus to the anus. It is a vast chemical and electrical warehouse of messages that influence not only the digestive system but every other cell and organ system in the body. There are 100 million enteric nerves in the small intestine alone, more than in the entire peripheral nervous system and equal to the number in the spinal cord. The number of enteric nerves in the large intestine have yet to be counted. Only 1,000-2,000 nerve fibers connect the human brain to the enteric system through the vagus nerve, therefore the gut's enteric nervous system functions priamarily on its own rather than being directed by the human brain. We think of nerve messages as electrical events so it is easy to think of 2000 telephone lines between the head and gut compared to 100 million telephone lines within the small intestine. The 2000 messages sent from the head will be heard but the dominant voices will be from the 100 million enteric telephone system's electrical messages.

The enteric nervous system controls the efficiency and effectiveness of gut functions. The gut's major function is to digest food, absorb the digested nutrients into the blood stream and defend against poisons. The enteric nervous system determines to a large extent what nutrients and how much of each is absorbed or excreted. It also sends messages to all other body organs via chemical messages.

A Chemical Messaging System

The enteric nervous system is a control system that sends its messages via chemicals as well as through electrical output. It produces information molecules that travel throughout the body to magnet sites on cells and organs. The same chemical messengers are produced by the enteric system and the brain. The "feel good" information molecules – endorphins, the "pain perception" information molecules – substance

P, the stress molecules – cortisol, and the calming information molecules – serotonin, are all produced in the gut's enteric nervous system and then travel to the rest of the body attaching to magnet sites and influencing function and behavior at that organ system site.

One of the most discussed information molecules in CPP is serotonin. Ninety five percent of the body's serotonin is produced in the gut not the brain! When the gut produces an abundance of serotonin it flows not only in the gut, influencing function there, but also to the head, the heart, the blood vessels, the uterus, and the bladder. What is serotonin's influence at these various sites? In the gut it facilitates contraction, in the heart it increases heart rate, in the blood vessels it stimulates constriction, in the uterus and bladder it induces contraction, in the head it facilitates sleep and decreases pain perception.

Another chemical messenger produced by the enteric nervous system is substance P whose influence is felt throughout the body. Substance P increases the perception of pain and heart rate and decreases blood pressure.

When Humpty Dumpty Falls...

The enteric nervous system in CPP often has difficulty maintaining a balance between rest and work. One illustrative example is the serotonin production in the enteric nervous system. The 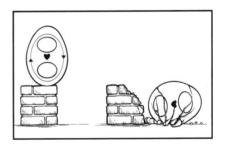 chemical messenger serotonin is released when there is pressure on the bowel lining cells. This serotonin excites peristalsis and thus elimination. If the release of serotonin is excessive then peristalsis is initially increased which causes diarrhea, dehydration and discomfort. As excessive serotonin production continues it "drowns" the gut's magnet receptor sites and as with any drowning victim the sites cease to function so the gut shuts down. This excessive serotonin results in paralysis of the gut until the excess serotonin is broken down or otherwise incapacitated. Constipation and even fecal impaction with inflammation is the result. Constipation and impaction of the gut is accompanied by abdominal pain, inability to stand up right and a shuffling gait with quick fatigue. In severe cases the individual cannot get up from a chair without help.

Another example of imbalance in chemical messengers produced by the enteric nervous system is the production of substance P. Substance P excites pain fibers that travel to the brain with information about pain and discomfort. When excessive substance P is present in the gut and spinal fluid, pain messages increase along the pain fibers. Additionally, the fibers that transmit other sensations like touch, pressure, heat, cold, sound and light can become highly sensitized and begin to transmit messages that are interpreted by the brain as pain rather than as touch, pressure or light sensation. Substance P has increased the body's pain sensitivity significantly without any major trauma having occurred.

An optimally functioning enteric division of the ANS stimulates efficient function of the heart, lungs, uterus, bladder, brain, pancreas, and liver, as well as the digestive system of the gut. When there is dysfunction or imbalance of the enteric system every other organ system is at risk for dysfunction as well. The enteric nervous system communicates with the heart via the vagus nerve complex, with the pancreas which produces insulin via enteric peripheral nerves and information chemicals, and with uterus and bladder much the same way. If the enteric nervous system is in a high activation mode the gut will transfer food from mouth to anus faster than usual. Additionally the uterus and the bladder could be more irritable, the heart could beat faster, and the pancreas could produce and dump increased amounts of insulin into the blood stream. The entire body is effected when the enteric nervous system of the gut is dysfunctional. When the dysfunctional chemical and electrical messaging system of the enteric nervous system is understood the gut becomes an essential focus of assessment and self care in the management of CPP symptoms.

Who Is The Boss?

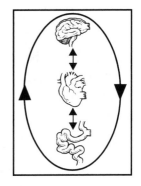

The head, heart and gut all have control centers described as both intrinsic and extrinsic. Intrinsic describes the ability to regulate their own organ system without external input. Extrinsic describes the ability to influence other organs and systems as well as their own. The ANS regulates the heart through the vagus nerve, a part of the parasympathetic division. The gut's enteric nervous system influences the heart through the same vagus nerve. This influence on the heart is significant but the heart also has its own intrinsic nervous system which keeps it functioning independent of outside control centers.

The heart will continue to beat in isolation just as the gut will continue to push food from the small intestine through the large intestine when there is no input from the human brain. Therefore symptoms of high heart rate, low blood pressure and abdominal pain are not necessarily mediated from the brain rather they can be greatly influenced by the heart's intrinsic control system "brain" and the gut's intrinsic control system (enteric) "brain."

The heart and gut's primary connection to the head is through the vagus nerve, an electrical messaging system. Messages from the brain to the heart and gut slows the heart rate and speeds up the gut peristalsis (rhythmical contractions). The enteric and cardiac control centers transmit messages to the brain via the vagus nerve informing and cajoling the brain centers in the head to provide necessary management of vital functions.

The heart, gut and head also communicate with each other via chemical messengers. These chemical messengers move through the blood stream to every cell of the body, finding body cells that have receptors and attract them like magnets. They attach and make significant changes in cell structure and organ function. Therefore, in CPP the dysfunctional messaging systems can be both electrical and/or chemical.

In the past focus of treatment has been primarily to alter the brain's function. Now we begin to look at the possible dysfunction in the heart and gut because they too direct other body functions in a significant way. As Melissa, 21, said to her physician, "This condition is manic depression of the body not the mind." She was describing the erratic, unpredictable behavior of the gut and heart control centers that resulted in her pain, fatigue, and other CPP symptoms. To better explain the influence on the whole body, take the example of the lungs and breathing.

The Last Breath....

One of the major functions of the head, heart and gut control centers is to regulate the breathing diaphragm which is essential for both life and health. The breathing diaphragm functions under ANS control expanding the lungs, filling them with oxygen and collapsing them to expel carbon dioxide. The breathing diaphragm does not have its own intrinsic nervous system so it cannot function in isolation from the head, heart and gut control centers. Rather it has dual innervation from the ANS and the voluntary nervous system. With ANS dysfunction, CPP individuals exhibit abnormal diaphragmatic breathing patterns. The breathing diaphragm action decreases and/or becomes shallow and ineffective. It is unable to automatically tighten and relax effectively, at times remaining in a semicontracted, tight state for long periods. This causes shortness of breath, chest, abdominal and back pain. Accessory muscles of the neck and upper chest take over much of the breathing activity. Breathing effectiveness and efficiency is compromised. The internal organs, i.e., stomach, liver, pancreas, intestines, bladder, uterus and bowel are all suspended from the breathing diaphragm either directly or indirectly by fascial "strings" so that with every breath the breathing diaphragm is gently, rhythmically moving the abdominal organs. The gentle movement of the internal organs with each breath is significantly decreased when accessory muscles take over breathing patterns. The breathing diaphragm is responsible for regulating the pH of every cell in the body – that is the acid-base balance of each cell. It also regulates the carbon dioxide-oxygen balance throughout the body – essentially bringing needed oxygen to the cells and getting rid of waste carbon dioxide. The body pH changes with accessory muscle breathing compared to diaphragmatic breathing. Twelve to fourteen times per minute each minute of each day every day of the year the breathing diaphragm performs this essential function, directed by the ANS.

All of these changes can be precipitated by dysfunctional head, heart and gut control centers and can lead to pain, fatigue, and associated symptoms of CPP.

The Reproductive Hormone Axis (RHA)

The Reproductive Hormone Axis includes the ovaries and uterus in females, the gonads in males, the adrenal glands and fat in both females and males. These organs produce both male and female chemical messengers composed of fats broken down into essential fatty acids. Females will produce more female hormones than male hormones and vice versa but both females and males produce female and male hormones. Female hormones include estrogen, progesterone, relaxin, and oxytocin. Testosterone is the most familiar male hormone.

Estrogen, Progesterone, and Testosterone

In females, estrogen and progesterone (chemical messengers) are produced primarily in the ovaries and effect all organ systems including the brain, the gut, and the muscles. (Figure 4)

A consideration in CPP symptoms is the ratio of estrogen/ progesterone to testosterone levels. Testosterone, the male hormone, facilitates muscle definition and strength, modifies pain perception, and alters the distribution of fat around the waistline. An imbalance in

---

Female Reproductive Hormone Function

Estrogen	Progesterone
increases blood pressure	decreases blood pressure
improves sleep	decreases digestive activity
increases well being	increases appetite
increases energy	increases sex drive
increases endorphins	increases water retention
increases serotonins	increases breast engorgement
increases brain blood flow	decreases well being
increases thyroid function	

Figure 4

the ratio of estrogen/progesterone to testosterone in females can aggravate muscle spasms and increase pain perception.

Daily, Monthly, Yearly Cycles

Estrogen and progesterone vary on a monthly/28 day cycle. They also vary during the year, the highest level in April through July and the lowest from October through January. When CPP individuals complain of increased symptoms during the winter months it may be that the estrogen/progesterone levels have fallen excessively, much like at the end of the monthly cycle. If increased symptoms occur in the spring it may be an over abundance of estrogen/progesterone. Supplementing with phytoestrogens/progesterones in natural food or cream form or using hormone replacement therapy on a temporary or permanent basis may assist the organ systems maintain and balance function. In a clinical trial, pain and fatigue, bowel, bladder and menstrual cycle dysfunction improved in a small group of women who used phytoestrogen and progesterone during the winter months and again in the spring.

Mary described becoming incapacitated with pain, fatigue, abdominal bloating and gut dysfunction around Thanksgiving every year. She would be in bed, unable to work or go to school. No dietary changes seemed to help. She would gradually recover over a 4-6 week period. Using the phytoestrogen and progesterone creams she was able to work and attend school. She did not become ill or need to limit her activities any more than other times of the year. She is now confident that her life is under better control and balance.

Hormone levels vary on a daily cycle in males. It is typical for the levels to cycle up to eight times a day. Each of these cycles has the potential to effect CPP symptoms particularly when there are imbalances or variations in the cycle.

RHA-HPA-ANS

The Leg Bone is Connected to the Hip Bone...

The reproductive hormones help to regulate the HPA (hypothalamic-pituitary-adrenal axis) and vice versa. During chronic stress, there is a decrease in function of both the HPA and the RHA. Individuals under chronic stress exhibit diminished reproductive capability as well as fatigue, sleep disruption and illness. If there is a dysregulation of the RHA there will likely be an associated dysregulation of the HPA axis. For example, if estrogen, a part of the RHA, is chronically elevated, the HPA axis may be significantly depressed. If RHA is in dysregulation the HPA opiods are decreased. Internally produced opiods are the natural analgesia in the body. Opioid receptors are present at all levels of the nervous system. Increased HPA axis dysregulation can increase the pain perception throughout the body. The ANS influences the HPA; the HPA influences the RHA; the RHA influences the ANS. The loop never ends and it can be affected at many junctions.

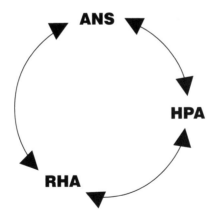

What is the Anatomy of Chronic Pelvic Pain and Low Back Pain?

Chapter 5

Anatomy and Function

Pelvic pain can originate from striated muscles. These muscles may elicit pelvic pain symptoms from trigger points, tender points, elevated resting tone or dysfunction during a contraction with secondary ischemia and/or irritation of associated structures. The striated muscles include:

breathing diaphragm

abdominals
{
    rectus abdominus
    internal/external obliques
    transverse abdominus

pyramidalis
iliopsoas
pectineus

adductors
{
    adductor longus
    adductor brevis
    adductor magnus

quadratus lumborum

gluteals
{
    gluteus maximus
    gluteus minimus
    gluteus medius

sphincters
{
    external anal sphincter
    external urinary sphincter

piriformis
gracilis
sartorius

deep external rotators $\left\{\begin{array}{l}\text{inferior \& superior gemelli}\\ \text{quadratus femoris}\\ \text{obturator internus}\end{array}\right.$

hamstrings   biceps femoris

pelvic diaphragm $\left\{\begin{array}{l}\text{pubococcygeus}\\ \text{iliococcygeus}\\ \text{puborectalis}\end{array}\right.$

urogenital diaphragm $\left\{\begin{array}{l}\text{transverse perineal}\\ \text{bulbospongeosus}\\ \text{ischiocavernus}\end{array}\right.$

coccygeus

Muscle · Location · Function · Pain Pattern

Breathing Diaphragm

Location – The breathing diaphragm attaches to ribs, sternum, and upper lumbar spine.

Function – The breathing diaphragm functions include:

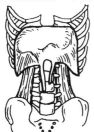

- oxygen/carbon dioxide exchange,
- Ph level determinant in all body cells,
- blood/lymph pump from lower body to heart,
- thoracic-lumbar spine mobilization,
- internal organ motility, mobility,
- sympathetic/parasympathetic nervous system balance.

Pain Pattern – Breathing diaphragm dysfunction leads to pain patterns in the head and neck, thoracic spine area, abdominal/chest region.

Abdominals

Rectus Abdominus

Location – The rectus abdominus attaches to the symphysis pubis distally and to the xyphoid process of the sternum and the costal cartilage of ribs 5, 6, 7.

Function – The rectus abdominus flexes the trunk and supports the internal organs.

Pain Pattern – The rectus abdominus refers pain to the back in a horizontal pattern between the scapular angle and the iliac crest. Pain in the lower right quadrant can imitate appendicitis. Dysmennorhea pain can be significantly increased from trigger points in the rectus abdominus.

Note- A non-painful condition known as rectus diastasis is separation of the fascia, called the linea alba, between the two rectus abdominus muscles. An excessive seperation decreases visceral organ support and can initiate abdominal trigger points.

Internal and External Obliques

Location-The internal and external oblique muscles attach to the ribs and costal cartilage proximally and the pubic bone, iliac crest, linea alba, and inguinal ligament distally.

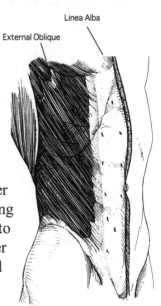

Linea Alba

External Oblique

Function – The oblique muscles rotate the trunk and flex the trunk depending which muscles are contracting.

Pain Pattern – The trigger points of the upper oblique muscles can lead to heartburn, belching and vomiting as well as pain in the mid to superior abdominal area. Lower oblique trigger points refer pain across the lower abdominal region to either side and can cause diarrhea.

Transverse Abdominus

Location – The transverse abdominus
attaches to fascia of the rectus abdominus,
inguinal ligament, the iliac crests,
thoracodorsal fascia, and the costal cartilage
of the lower six ribs extending into the
breathing diaphragm. It is the deepest of the
abdominal muscles.

Function – The transverse abdominus functions
to support the abdominal viscera, the low back and
the sacroiliac joint. In conjunction with other muscles
it works much like a girdle.

Pyramidalis

Location – The pyramidalis superior attachment is to the linea alba
midway between the umbilicus and the pubis and its distal attachment
is to the symphysis pubis, blending with the transverse abdominus,
obliques and adductor attachments over the symphysis pubis.

Function – The pyramidalis functions to stabilize the symphysis
pubis joint and to support the lower abdominal viscera.

Pain Pattern – The trigger points of the pyramidalis are superior to
the pubic symphysis and the pain pattern extends to the umbilicus.

Iliopsoas

Location – The psoas muscle attaches to the
vertebral bodies and transverse processes of T12-
L5, to the diaphragm and blends distally with the
iliacus. The iliacus attaches on the inner aspect of
the iliac fossa, sacroiliac joint, and sacrum. There
is distal attachment to the lesser trochanter and
joint capsule of the anterior femur.

Function – The iliopsoas functions to flex the
trunk on the hip and flex the hip on the trunk.

Pain Pattern – The trigger points of the
iliopsoas refer pain vertically up the back from
below the iliac crest and anteriorly from the

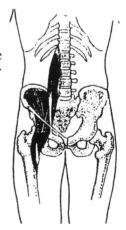

anterior superior iliac spine into the groin and anterior thigh. The CPP posture is pelvic anterior tilt, hip flexion, and increased lumbar lordosis, a posture indicative of iliopsoas dysfunction.

Pectineus

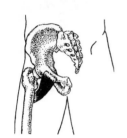

Location – The pectineus attaches to the superior aspect of the pubic rami and the anterior, superior femur.

Function – The pectineus adducts and flexes the femur on the pelvis.

Pain Pattern – Trigger points of the pectineus refer pain deep in the groin and into the anterior medial thigh. It is often described as a deep ache.

Adductors – Magnus, Longus, Brevis

Location – The adductor muscles attach proximally to the pubic rami and ischial tuberosity and distally to the shaft and medial condyle of the femur.

Function – The adductor muscles adduct the femur on the hip and anteriorly or posteriorly rotate the pelvis in standing.

Pain Pattern – Trigger points of the adductors refer pain deep into the pelvic region, proximally into the groin, and distally towards the knee. The pelvic pain is felt around the pubis, vagina, rectum, and bladder.

Quadratus Lumborum

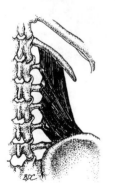

Location – The quadratus lumborum attaches proximally to the 12th rib and transverse processes of the upper four lumbar vertebrae and distally to the iliac crest, iliolumbar ligament and fourth and fifth lumbar transverse processes.

Function – The quadratus lumborum elevates the hip and assists in stabilizing the lumbosacral junction.

Pain Pattern – Trigger points of the quadratus refer pain along the ipsilateral lumbar spine, from the sacrum to the inferior buttocks and laterally along the inferior aspect of the iliac crest.

Gluteals – Maximus, Medius, Minimus

Location – The gluteals attach proximally along the external aspect of the iliac crest and the sacrum. Distally they attach to the gluteal tuberosity of the femur and iliotibial band.

Function – The gluteal muscles abduct, externally rotate and extend the hip.

Pain Pattern – Trigger points of the gluteals refer pain into the sacral and buttocks areas. Pain can be referred down the lateral leg even below the knee.

Sphincters - External Anal, External Urinary

Location – The external sphincters are circular muscle surrounding the anal and urinary outlets.

Function – The external sphincters function like purse strings pulling shut to maintain closure of the anus and urethra.

Pain Pattern – Trigger points of the external sphincters refer pain into the pelvis in the area of the rectum and anus, urethra, bladder and vagina. There can be

External Anal Sphincter

complaints of painful intercourse, bowel movements, and urination.

Piriformis

Location – The piriformis attaches proximally to the inner surface of the medial sacrum with distal attachment to the posterior aspect of the greater trochanter.

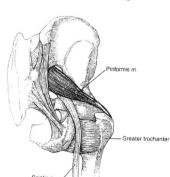

Piriformis m.

Greater trochanter

Sciatic n.

Function – The piriformis externally rotates the hip. In standing, it moves the sacrum on the pelvis.

Pain Pattern – The trigger points of the piriformis refer pain to the lower sacrum, buttocks, and posterior thigh.

Gracilis

Location – The gracilis attaches proximally to the pubic ramus and attaches distally to the tibia.

Function – The gracilis adducts and flexes the hip.

Pain Pattern – Trigger points of the gracilis refer pain to the groin.

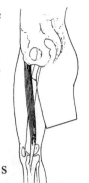

Sartorius

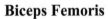

Location – The sartorius attaches proximally to the anterior superior iliac spine and distally to the medial tibia.

Function – The sartorius flexes and externally rotates the hip and flexes the knee.

Pain Pattern – Trigger points of the sartorius refer sharp tingling pain into the groin. It can participate in the entrapment of the lateral femoral cutaneous nerve leading to numbness along the lateral thigh.

Biceps Femoris

Location – The biceps femoris attaches proximally to the ischial tuberosity and sacrotuberous ligament. It attaches distally to the proximal posterior fibula.

Function – The biceps femoris extends the hip and flexes the knee.

Pain Pattern – Trigger points of the biceps femoris refer pain to the posterior thigh, buttocks and sacroiliac joint.

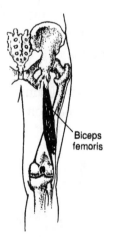

Biceps femoris

Deep Short Lateral Rotator Muscles
Inferior and Superior Gemelli, Quadratus Femoris

Location – The proximal attachment is to the medial aspect of the ischium and the distal attachment is to the greater trochanter.

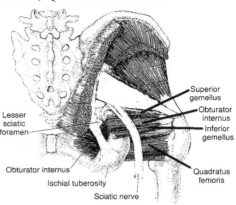

Function – The short rotator muscles laterally rotate the hip.

Pain Pattern – Trigger points are a source of deep hip and buttocks' pain.

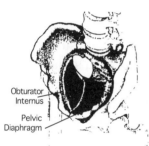

Obturator Internus
Location – The obturator internus attaches proximally covering the obturator foramen and blending with the arcuate tendon and distally to the greater trochanter.

Function – The obturator internus laterally rotates the hip and lifts the bladder, bowel and uterus into a functional position while assisting in closure of the urethra and anus.

Pain Pattern – Trigger points of the obturator internus refer pain into the deep pelvic region.

Pelvic Diaphragm/ Levator Ani
Pubococcygeus, Ileococcygeus, Puborectalis muscles

Location – The pelvic diaphragm attaches to the symphysis pubis, side walls of the ischium, blends with the arcuate tendon and via fascia/ ligaments to the sacrum and coccyx.

Function – The pelvic diaphragm supports the bladder, bowel and uterus in a functional position and assists in closure of the bladder and bowel outlet. It moves the sacrum on the pelvis.

Pain Pattern – Trigger points of the pelvic diaphragm refer pain to deep pelvic organs.

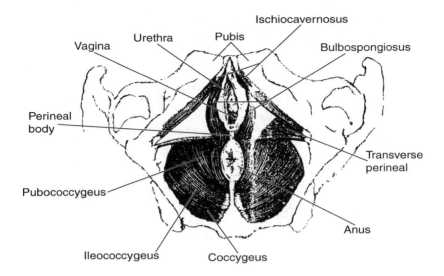

Labels: Ischiocavernosus, Vagina, Urethra, Pubis, Bulbospongiosus, Perineal body, Transverse perineal, Pubococcygeus, Anus, Ileococcygeus, Coccygeus

Urogenital Diaphragm/Perineal Muscles

Transverse Perineal, Ischiocavernus, Bulbospongiosus muscles

Location – The urogenital diaphragm muscles attach to the ischial tubererosity, pubic rami and perineal body.

Function – The urogenital diaphragm functions primarily to pump blood into the clitoris and penis. It facilitates closure of the urethra for short periods of time.

Pain Pattern – Trigger points of the urogenital diaphragm refer pain to the proximal one third of the vagina and superficial area around the urethral opening.

Coccygeus

Location – The coccygeus attaches to the sacrospinous ligament and the coccyx.

Function – The coccygeus is called the tail wagging muscle. It moves the sacrum/coccyx on the pelvis.

Pain Pattern – Trigger points of the coccygeus refer pain to the region around the anus and rectum.

Pelvic Fascia

The pelvic fascia surrounds the cervix of the uterus and attaches to the sacrum and pelvic walls. It extends out like spokes on a wheel incorporating support for the bladder, uterus, and bowel. It consists of collagen, elastin and muscle tissue so has contractile capabilities. In females it is estrogen dependent. Nerves and blood vessels run through the fascia to their end organs. (Figure 5)

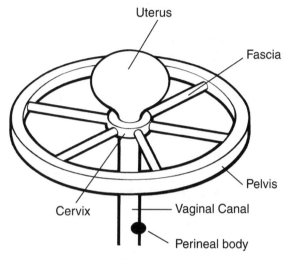

Figure 5 Pelvic Fascia

The Muscles of the Bladder and Urethra

The bladder is composed of relatively unorganized interdigitating longitudinal, horizontal, and oblique smooth muscle. The bladder outlet is circular muscle externally and longitudinal muscle internally. The body of the bladder expands to allow urine to accumulate. The bladder outlet's circular muscle remains closed to hold the urine in. Several times a day the body of the bladder contracts and the bladder outlet relaxes to let urine flow out. (Figure 6) The urethra is lined with smooth muscle.

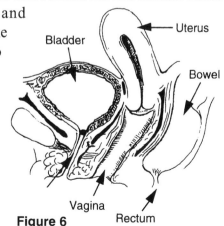

Figure 6

The Muscles of the Bowel, Rectum, and Anus

The intestines, small and large, are composed of a "tube within a tube" of smooth muscle. The smooth muscle tubes contract to propel the nutrients through the system, to facilitate the body's absorption of nutrients and water and to eliminate waste products.

Contraction frequency in the colon is approximately 6 cycles per second. The distal end of the intestines is the rectum and anus. Feces collect in the rectum while the anorectal angle is maintained by the puborectalis muscle. When pressure builds up in the rectum the anorectal angle straightens with relaxation of the puborectalis loops and the feces can descend. The internal anal sphincter automatically relaxes with increased pressure in the rectum. The external anal sphincter, under vuluntary control, contracts to hold feces in until the individual reaches the toilet.

The Muscles of the Uterus and Vagina

The uterus is composed of three layers of smooth muscle – longitudinal, oblique and circular. The body of the uterus is 3-4 inches long, and composed primarily of longitudinal and oblique muscle fibers. The outlet of the uterus is called the cervix and has a higher concentration of circular muscle. The vagina is lined with smooth muscle except for the distal one third which contains striated muscle.

Chapter 6

Pelvic Muscle Force Field Anatomy and Innervation

Muscles of the Pelvic Muscle Force Field

The Pelvic Muscle Force Field (PMFF) is the rotator cuff musculature of the pelvis forming the most inferior basic support structure for the internal abdominal organs and lumbo-sacral region of the spine.

The PMFF is composed of a series of striated muscles innervated by the voluntary and autonomic nervous systems. The PMFF is contained within the lower pelvis and finds its support and many of its major attachments on pelvic bone structure. Besides bony attachments, another major attachment for the PMFF is the arcuate/obturator tendon (referred to as the arcuate tendon). The arcuate tendon attaches anteriorly near the symphysis pubis and posteriorly to the ischial spine bilaterally. The obturator internus and pelvic diaphragm muscles attach to this tendon. The urethropelvic ligament and the periurethral fascia blend with the arcuate tendon.

The PMFF first described by Hulme includes the following muscles:

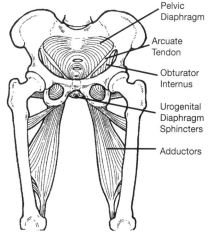

      Obturator internus
      Pelvic diaphragm
         (levator ani)
      Urogenital diaphragm
      External urinary and anal
         sphincters
      Hip adductors (Figure 7)

Figure 7: Pelvic Muscle Force Field

The obturator internus muscle attaches within the pelvis along the lateral aspect of the arcuate tendon and substantially covers the obturator foramen attaching around its border. It exits the pelvis at a 120° angle around the lesser sciatic notch and attaches to the posterior superior aspect of the greater trochanter of the femur.

Typically, the obturator internus muscle is described as an outward rotator of the hip when the hip is in relative extension. With the hip flexed, the obturator internus outwardly rotates and abducts the hip. Another function of the obturator internus is support through the PMFF of the internal abdominal organs of bladder, uterus and bowel.

The pelvic diaphragm (levator ani) attaches within the pelvis to the medial aspect of the arcuate tendons bilaterally, to anterior, posterior and lateral aspects of the lower pelvis and to the sacrum and coccyx. The pelvic diaphragm is composed of the pubococcygeus, the iliococcygeus, and the puborectalis muscles. These muscles run in a sling-like fashion from the symphysis pubis, pubic rami, and ischium on one side to unite with fibers from the opposite side and then to connective tissue attaching to the sacrum and coccyx posteriorly.

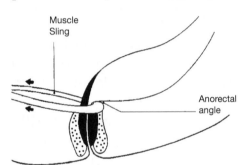

Sling's Resting Tone.

The pelvic diaphragm muscle has a preponderance of slow twitch, type I muscle fibers. It functions much like a postural muscle of the peripheral skeleton, maintaining relatively high resting tone. This resting tone helps maintain the anorectal and bladder angles necessary for bowel and bladder continence 24 hours a day. (Figure 8)

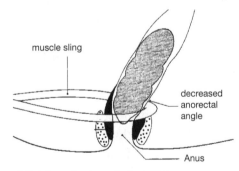

Inhibition during defecation.

Figure 8: Pelvic Diaphragm Sling resting tone and during defecation

During urination the pelvic diaphragm slings must relax/release to allow urine to pass through the urethra. When having a bowel movement the pelvic diaphragm slings release to allow feces to pass through the rectum. The pelvic diaphragm does have its own rest/work cycle throughout daily life even though it is termed an endurance or postural muscle rather than a sprinter muscle.

The urethropelvic ligament is thickened fascial fibers that envelop the bladder neck and proximal urethra and extend laterally across the levator ani to the arcuate tendon bilaterally. This ligament transfers forces from the pulley system of the obturator internus and arcuate tendon to facilitate elevation and support of the proximal bladder neck/ urethra.

The urogenital diaphragm/perineum muscle group is positioned in the anterior two thirds of the region between the symphysis pubis and coccyx. It attaches to the symphysis pubis, pubic rami, perineal body, and ischial tuberosities. The muscles that form the urogenital diaphragm include the deep transverse perineal interconnected by fascial planes with the external urethral sphincter. In some references the bulbospongiosus and ischiocavernus muscles are also included in the urogenital diaphragm muscle group. This group of muscles interdigitates via fascia and connective tissue with the pelvic diaphragm and via the perineal body with the external anal sphincter.

The urogenital diaphragm has a preponderance of fast twitch, type II muscle fibers, which contract quickly and forcefully but also fatigues relatively quickly. The urogenital diaphragm function in maintaining continence is to close the urethra distal to the bladder outlet. The fibers reflexively close the urethra during stress, e.g.. coughing or sneezing. The fatigue factor of the urogenital diaphragm's fibers does not allow them to effectively function in endurance postural occlusion during daily activities except as part of the PMFF.

The adductor longus and brevis muscles attach to the medial aspect of the femur and to the pubic rami adjacent to the urogenital diaphragm attachment. There is no evidence that adductor fibers interdigitate with urogenital or pelvic diaphragm fibers. They adduct and inwardly rotate the femur on the pelvis. These adductors function as part of the PMFF through the structural connection to the femur. They facilitate active pelvic and urogenital diaphragm contraction. At the completion of the PMFF "obturator action" phase the obturator internus muscles are in a contracted and shortened position. The adductors function to relengthen the obturator internus muscles during the "adductor action" phase. At completion of "adductor action" phase the femurs are adducted and the obturator internus muscles lengthened. Then the "obturator action" phase can begin again with the relengthened obturator internus muscles doing most of the work.

The adductors are not attached directly to the urogenital and pelvic diaphragm muscles, so when they contract there is no direct caudal force exerted on the PMFF. Rather, the femur position is changed during the adductor contraction, which lengthens the obturators via the femoral attachment. The adductor muscles also facilitate action of the urogenital and pelvic diaphragm muscles through proprioceptive neuromuscular facilitation principles via the close approximation of their attachment to the urogenital and pelvic diaphragm muscle attachments on the pubic bone. Again, there is no caudal direction of force, because there is no direct interdigitation between the muscle groups.

The pelvic diaphragm and urogenital diaphragm are not isolated muscles that attach from bone to bone contracting to move one bone on another bone through a joint action. There is that component at the sacrococcygeal and sacroiliac joints, but this is not there primary function. These striated muscles are present to support the bladder, uterus and bowel and to facilitate continence, appropriate elimination and sexual and reproductive activity throughout the life span. Their structural attachments are as much muscle to fascia to tendon to muscle to ligament to other muscle as they are bone to bone. As such, they form a dynamic pelvic muscle force field, not a pelvic floor.

In summary, the PMFF functions with a rhythmical balance of rest/ work cycles involving the prime movers of obturator internus and adductors and the organ support muscle being the pelvic diaphragm (levator ani) in conjunction with the urogenital diaphragm and external sphincters. These muscles function as an interdigitated and interrelated synergistic unit, not as separate entities in the support of abdominal organs, in stabilization of the lumbo-pelvic and sacroiliac region, and in reflexive action for continence.

Innervation of the Pelvic Muscle Force Field

The voluntary nervous system innervation of the PMFF is from sacral roots 2, 3, 4 via the pudendal and pelvic nerves. An individual uses this system to accomplish hip motion during daily activities and when holding urine or a bowel movement while he/she rushes to the bathroom. Most of the day the PMFF resting tone is influenced primarily by the ANS. The resting tone of all striated muscle, including the PMFF, is largely determined by the muscle spindle's gamma bias within each muscle fiber bundle. That muscle spindle is innervated primarily by the sympathetic portion, thoracic 10, 11, 12 and lumbar 1, 2, of the ANS ganglion chain.

Therefore, the resting tone of the pelvic and urogenital diaphragm muscles is, to a great extent, determined by the ANS. When resting tone of the PMFF is elevated, back and pelvic pain and dysfunctional voiding are the usual symptoms, along with pain during intercourse and constipation. To effectively resolve high pelvic muscle resting tone, ANS training through Physiological Quieting is necessary.

Chapter 7

Pelvic Muscle Force Field Function

Function of the Bladder and Urethra

Most everyone wants to be dry and pain-free while carrying out daily activities and while sleeping at night. To accomplish that:
- the bladder must be happy, content and quiet while filling,
- the bladder outlet must be closed, and
- this must be accomplished without having to consciously think about it.

The bladder is composed of smooth muscle that is grumpy by nature. If it had its way it would push urine out as it flowed in throughout the day. An individual would have the choice of having wet pants most of the day or sitting on the toilet instead of a chair while doing his/her daily activities. What helps to keep the bladder quiet and happy until it is full?
- The autonomic nervous system continually sends soothing messages via the parasympathetic division to the bladder wall to keep it happy and content.
- Any PMFF contraction sends reflex messages to the bladder wall to be quiet and content. The reflex inhibition principle is in effect between the PMFF and the bladder.

These actions enable the bladder to fill with urine and wait 3-4 hours before telling the brain it is time to go to the bathroom. Twenty-four hours of the day the ANS is working to keep the bladder contented and quiet. An individual usually spends a minute or two 4-5 times/day toileting. So 5-10 minutes of each day the bladder gets to be grumpy and push urine out.

The outlet of the bladder is called the urethra. It is a tube that is squeezed shut 24 hours/day. It opens only the few minutes that bladder emptying occurs. What helps to keep the urethra closed all day while an individual jumps, runs, bends, sneezes, coughs, sits, or sleeps?

- The urethra is richly lined with blood vessels and mucous glands. The lining is sticky with mucous and other fluids to help keep it closed. This closure is called coaptation.
- The urethra is also lined with smooth muscle. The relatively high resting tone of this smooth muscle via the sympathetic division of the ANS maintains the urethra in a closed position.
- The bladder outlet is closed by the PMFF resting tone, which is relatively high. The resting tone of the slings maintains the bladder angle to keep the bladder outlet closed. Think of water in a straw. If the straw is bent the water stays in the straw because the PMFF maintains the bladder angle with the urethra. If the straw is straight the water runs out. That would be the PMFF slings more relaxed/released than its normal resting tone.
- The PMFF closes the outlet when the obturator internus and adductor muscles are active during daily activities or exercise.
- The slings of the pelvic diaphragm tighten to close the outlet when the obturators are active.
- The slings of the pelvic diaphragm tighten when the adductor muscles are active.
- When the adductor muscles are active and the legs move together there is some additional mechanical closing of the bladder outlet.

Holding urine in the bladder is a major job accomplished through urethral muscle resting tone, PMFF resting tone, multiple muscle action mechanisms of the PMFF, and mucosal coaptation of the urethra.

Releasing urine is accomplished through inhibition of ANS input to the bladder, bladder outlet, urethra, and PMFF. The parasympathetic input to the bladder wall is inhibited to allow the bladder wall to contract to push urine out. The sympathetic input to the bladder outlet is inhibited to allow the bladder outlet to open. The sympathetic input to the PMFF muscle spindles is inhibited to allow the pelvic diaphragm loops to relax to open the urethra.

Pelvic Muscle Force Field Function

The PMFF supports the lumbo-sacral region and the internal abdominal organs. It functions as an integral part of the urogenital continence system to maintain bladder and bowel continence and allow for effective and efficient elimination. It functions as an important hip stabilizer unit in standing posture and ambulation.

To better understand how the PMFF functions, quickly visualize:

The Bowl. The bowl is made of slings that run obliquely from front to back, forming the bottom and sidewalls of the bowl. There are 2-3 holes in the bottom of the bowl.

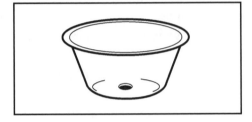

The Clothesline. An old-fashioned clothesline is made of two uprights and two clothes lines. A sheet is attached between the two clotheslines and also attached to the two uprights. There are pulley ropes attached to the two clotheslines that are stabilized in the ground. When the day is very windy the lady of the house tightens the outrigger pulleys which pulls the clotheslines laterally and raises the sheet up.

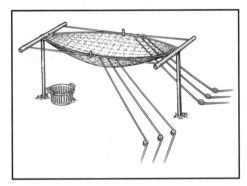

The Teeter Totter.

Two individuals of equal weight sit on the teeter totter and it is balanced. When the teeter totter is balanced each end is at the same level. When one of the individuals eats too many ice cream cones she weighs more than the other and the teeter totter is no longer balanced. One side tips up and the other tips down.

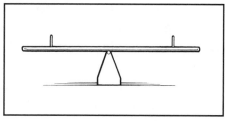

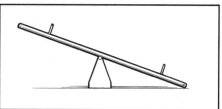

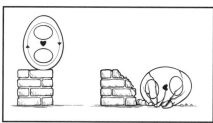

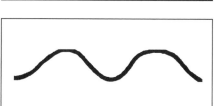

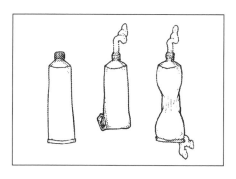

The Egg. An egg like Humpty Dumpty sits on a wall. When the egg is balanced it stays on the wall. When it is imbalanced it falls off the wall and breaks to pieces.

The Wave. An ocean wave moves in and out, up and down forever moving in rhythm coming in toward shore and going out with the tide. Everything that goes up must come down.

The Toothpaste Tube. A toothpaste tube can be squeezed from the bottom up, from the middle, or from the top down. The toothpaste would be squeezed up and out the top when squeezed from the bottom up. When squeezed from the middle the toothpaste would be pushed towards both ends. When squeezed from the top the toothpaste would be pushed to the bottom and out any holes or weakened areas.

Now we can correlate these everyday visuals with PMFF function.

The core of the PMFF is the **bowl**. It is the pelvic diaphragm, a series of muscle slings that run obliquely from the front to the back of the pelvis. The slings attach in the front and sides to the pubic bone and the ileum. The slings attach via ligament and fascia at the back of the pelvis to the sacrum and coccyx. At the bottom of the slings are 2 openings in males and 3 openings in females, the vaginal opening, urethral and anal openings. These muscle slings have resting tone that is relatively high and maintains the shape of the bowl at all times. The resting tone of the bowl is termed postural tone. It maintains closure of the openings at the bottom of the bowl so nothing leaks out.

The pelvic diaphragm is interdigitated with the urogenital diaphragm and external sphincters. They function in conjunction with the pelvic diaphragm to close the urethra.

The pelvic diaphragm core is interdigitated with the obturator internus via the arcuate tendon much like the sheet is attached to the outrigger pulleys via the **clothesline**. The sheet is the pelvic diaphragm, the outrigger pulleys are the obturator internus muscles attached to the ground (the femurs), and the clotheslines are the arcuate tendons. When the outrigger pulleys shorten, the clotheslines are pulled outward and the sheet is elevated keeping the openings at the bottom of the sheet/bowl closed.

The PMFF function includes alternating action of obturator internus and adductor muscles like a **teeter-totter.** If the bowl is the center of the teeter-totter, the obturator internus muscles and the adductor muscles are the individuals on each end of the teeter-totter. The obturator and adductor muscles alternately contract tipping the ends up and down but the central core maintains a stable supported position. The obturator muscles contract to lift and maintain the bowl in position. The adductor muscles contract to lengthen the obturator muscles after their contraction phase. The adductor muscles contract to send electrical overflow into the bowl to keep it in a stable supported and closed position.

The PMFF acts synergistically with the transverse abdominus, mutifidus and lumbo-pelvic fascia like the **Humpty Dumpty egg** balanced on the wall. When the PMFF contracts there is synergistic contraction of the transverse abdominus and vice versa. The transverse abdominus contraction tightens the lumbo-pelvic fascia and facilitates multifidus contraction to support the low back and internal organs. When the ratio of PMFF contraction and transverse abdominus contraction is optimal **Humpty Dumpty** is balanced and functional. If the abdominal muscles, especially the obliques and rectus abdominus, contract excessively **Humpty Dumpty** is imbalanced, and crashes to the ground in many pieces.

The top of the **Humpty Dumpty egg** is the breathing diaphragm. It functions much like an **ocean wave**. The breathing diaphragm moves up and down 12-14 times per minute. As the breathing diaphragm moves down with inhale intra-abdominal pressure increases and tends to push the bladder down putting pressure on the outlets of the bowl. The PMFF must maintain its position and support of the bladder, bowel, and lumbar spine to counteract this increased pressure. It accomplishes this by lifting with the outrigger pulleys (obturators) and facilitating action of the bowl (pelvic diaphragm) through overflow of electrical activity from the adductors. On exhale the breathing diaphragm returns to a dome shape elevating the bladder as much as 1-3 cm. and decreasing intra-abdominal pressure. The PMFF can be at relative rest during the exhale phase if there are no outside factors that increase intra-abdominal pressure. When there are outside forces that increase intra-abdominal pressure, the PMFF can use adductor muscles to increase the lift force of the pelvic diaphragm.

The PMFF, abdominals, and breathing diaphragm work together like pushing on a **toothpaste tube**. When the transverse abdominus and PMFF are synergistically contracting during exhale, the toothpaste (internal organs) is pushed from the bottom up towards the top of the tube. When the oblique abdominals are contracted from the top down as in a curl up or crunch, the toothpaste tube is squeezed from the top or middle pushing the toothpaste down and out the bottom of the tube. It is important to use muscles appropriately in support of the lumbar spine and internal organs in order to have optimal health and function. In otherwords it is important to have the toothpaste pushed from the bottom of the tube up.

The pelvic muscle force field is integral to optimal pain-free function of the:
- Low back and pelvis during daily activities,
- Lumbosacral region during upright posture, balance and gait

• Urogenital system in maintaining continence.

The pelvic muscle force field is integral to optimal pain-free function after:

- Spinal Surgery
- Hip Surgery
- Abdominal Surgery
- Knee Surgery
- Stroke
- Multiple Sclerosis
- Parkinson's Disease
- Head Injury.

Chapter 8

Breathing Diaphragm, Abdominal, Back and Foot Musculature

Breathing Diaphragm and Trunk Musculature in Relation to the PMFF

The breathing diaphragm, abdominals (particularly transverse abdominus), latisimus dorsi, gluteals, and multifidus are integral muscles in optimal PMFF function. They are not directly part of the PMFF but function in an integrated system of support and facilitate bladder and bowel function, lumbosacral stability, balance and ambulation.

The breathing diaphragm rests in a dome shape at the top of the abdomen attached to ribs, sternum and lumbar spine. In diaphragmatic breathing, the diaphragm descends and returns to the rest position 12-14 times per minute each minute of each day. This action helps maintain the optimal pH of all body fluids and optimal oxygen-carbon dioxide balance. It gently mobilizes the thoracic and lumbar spine 12-14 times per minute. In addition to these important factors, the breathing diaphragm movement massages the sympathetic nerve roots as they exit the thoracic and upper lumbar vertebrae. It functions as a pump for blood and lymph circulation within the pelvic organs and related structures. The major organs of the trunk are suspended from the diaphragm either directly or indirectly so the rhythmical movement of the diaphragm helps maintain normal mobility of these organs, and lifts the bladder 2-3 cm during the exhalation phase of breathing. There is evidence that the breathing diaphragm in conjunction with the transverse abdominus assists in spinal stabilization by increasing the intra-abdominal pressure during limb movement according to Richardson et al. There is evidence of synergistic contraction of the breathing diaphragm, transverse abdominus, and pelvic diaphragm muscles, as described by Hodges and Richardson. Diaphragmatic breathing is essential for spinal health, bladder and bowel health and continence. Diaphragm breathing is the first exercise to implement in order to achieve spinal and bowel/bladder health.

Breathing diaphragm movement is directly related to abdominal tone and contraction. As the breathing diaphragm descends, it compresses the abdominal contents, which are pushed down and toward the openings in the pelvic musculature, or up and out, expanding the abdominal cavity slightly in an anterior and lateral direction. If the abdominal muscles are forcefully contracting during the inhale phase of diaphragmatic breathing the force is directed down and out through the pelvic muscle openings of the urethra, vagina, and anus. If the abdominal muscles are actively contracting during the inhale phase of diaphragmatic breathing, the diaphragm hits a metaphorical brick wall. Unable to complete its normal descent breathing is performed by the upper chest and neck accessory muscles. During the exhale phase of diaphragmatic breathing the diaphragm ascends. The transverse abdominus, is synergistcally activiated during pursed lip exhale and can increase the force of the exhale. In older adults who are consistently "waiting to exhale", this can be a very beneficial pattern of movement. Inhale, abdominals relax; exhale with pursed lips, abdominals, specifically transverse abdominus, automatically contracts.

The relationship between the pelvic and the abdominal muscles is of importance in maintaining continence. In preliminary results, Sapsford et. al. describe that gentle activation of the transverse abdominus facilitated action of the pubococcygeus, and gentle activation of the obliques facilitated action of the iliococcygeus and ischiococcygeus. Puborectalis action was associated with rectus abdominus contraction. The oblique abdominal muscles are primarily phasic muscles, according to Richardson and Jull, and coordinate activation with the contralateral adductor muscles, as reported by

Snijders et. al. The transverse abdominus acts more as a postural muscle and assists in trunk stabilization, according to Hodges and Richardson. It is active even with gentle pelvic muscle contraction. The transverse abdominus is considered a respiratory muscle during extended exhalation, as well as a postural stabilization muscle, according to Richardson et. al.

Coordinating the breathing diaphragm and abdominal muscle action with effective PMFF activity is the ultimate goal. The exhale phase of diaphragmatic breathing coordinates well with transverse abdominus tightening and the adductor action phase of PMFF contraction. In other words, during exhale, abdominal muscles tighten, legs roll in, and the pelvic and urogenital diaphragm muscles contract.

Vleeming et. al. describe the interconnection of the latissimus dorsi muscle and the contralateral gluteus maximus via the thoracodorsal fascia. In function this oblique system is effective in stabilizing the back and sacroiliac joint and transferring load during rotational activities, as reported by Mooney. In theory, the latissimus dorsi and the gluteus maximus coordinate with the obturator internus of the PMFF to stabilize the sacrum and coccyx at the base of this internal chain.

As the diaphragm descends with inhale, the latissimus dorsi and gluteals gently contract with the obturator action phase of PMFF contraction. The inhale phase of diaphragmatic breathing coordinates effectively with external rotation of the shoulder, external rotation of the hips, and abdominal release to allow the diaphragm descent. The pelvic and urogenital diaphragm muscles are passively elevated through the pulley system of the force field, and facilitation of their active contraction is through overflow from the obturator internus muscle contraction. In summary, the breathing diaphragm and trunk musculature act synergistically with the PMFF in daily function.

Foot Musculature in Relation to the PMFF

Intrinsic foot muscle function is coordinated with pelvic muscle function via striated muscle innervation from sacral nerve roots 2, 3, 4 & 5. These nerve roots are responsible for innervation of the external urethral and anal sphincters, the pelvic and urogenital diaphragm, the obturator internus, and the gluteal and foot intrinsic muscles. The human embryo reabsorbs the tail during weeks 5 and 6. During this caudal regression process, asymmetrical or symmetrical neuronal loss may occur effecting sacral roots 2, 3, 4 & 5 due to this shared innervation. It is common that motor deficits in the feet can be correlated with dysfunction in the PMFF. Asymmetrical or symmetrical inability to abduct the toes or intrinsic muscle atrophy in the feet can indicate pelvic muscle dysfunction with neurological origin, as described by Galloway.

Intrinsic foot musculature is interconnected with the PMFF via fascial planes. The PMFF interconnects with the sacrotuberous ligament, which connects to the biceps femoris (hamstring), which interdigitates via fascia with the posterior tibialis and peroneal muscles, which have fascial links to the foot intrinsic muscles. In theory, strengthening the intrinsic foot muscles and stimulating sensory nerve fibers in the foot can improve the muscle function of the PMFF. Abnormal gait and standing posture can contribute to significant pelvic muscle dysfunction and vice versa.

In summary the foot musculature functions synergistically with the PMFF.

The Toothpaste Tube

The toothpaste tube is composed of the toothpaste – internal organs bladder, intestines, stomach, liver, pancreas, uterus, and ovaries encased in a container formed of:

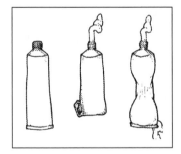

1. the PMFF
2. the abdominals
    a. the obliques
    b. the rectus abdominus
    c. the tranverse abdominus
3. the erector spinae
4. the multifidus
5. the breathing diaphragm

The toothpaste can be pushed from the bottom up, from the top down, or from the middle.

When the toothpaste is pushed from the top down the pressure eventually breaks down the base of the tube and the toothpaste squirts out the bottom. An individual with a chronic cough or sneeze, or who is constantly straining with breath holding is pushing the toothpaste from the top down. The breathing diaphragm and upper abdominal muscles are pushing the toothpaste from the top down. Eventually the individual experiences back pain, loss of urine and/or feces, and descent of the internal organs of bladder, bowel and uterus.

When the toothpaste is pushed from the middle of the tube some of the paste goes down and some is pushed up. The individual who does 200 crunches a day, or who does diagonal curl ups is pushing the toothpaste tube from the top and the middle using the oblique and rectus abdominus muscles. His/her waist gets smaller, the front of the tube gets tighter from the middle in both directions, and the toothpaste – the bladder, bowel, and uterus experience increased downward pressure. There are costs and benefits in the long and short term. In the short run the individual appears more attractive and has a smaller waist, and the low back is supported. However, there are long term costs. The organs experience repetitive downward pressure so the individual eventually may experience back pain, loss of urine and/or feces, and descent of the internal organs of bladder, bowel and uterus.

When the toothpaste is pushed from the bottom of the tube up all of the paste goes up. The individual who walks to work, and who has a balanced life of physical activity and rest uses muscles that push the toothpaste from the bottom up. With every step he/she takes the PMFF is activated in a balanced manor. This supports the closure of the bladder and bowel, gently maintains organ support in the pelvis and supports the lumbosacral spine in an optimal and functional position. The PMFF and transverse abdominus muscles push the toothpaste from the bottom up.

Staying dry and pain-free is best accomplished when the toothpaste tube is pushed from the bottom up more often than from the top down or the middle in both directions. All muscles are used for function in many different ways. Our culture and life-style has minimized the bottom up push of the tube and emphasized the top down and the middle in both directions to the detriment of bladder and bowel health and low back pain.

Chapter 9

Lumbo-Pelvic Stability, Balance and Ambulation

Stability of the lumbo-pelvic region is important because of the need to repetitively transfer weight, movement and force of the upper body through this region to the legs and feet. Stability implies the ability to effectively transmit weight, movement and force through joint structure. Stability of the lumbo-pelvic region has been conceptualized by Panjabi as three fold:

- passive – ligamentous/osteoarticular
- active – muscle/fascia
- control– neural

Stability is accomplished through the neutral zone which is a small range of movement on either side and through the neutral joint position where there is the least resistance of bony or ligamentous structures.

The passive – ligamentous/osteoarticular component of stability includes:

- the shape and cartilage of the sacroiliac, symphysis pubis, and lumbosacral joints
- the ligaments supporting the sacroiliac joint including:
  - iliolumbar ligament
  - sacrospinous ligament
  - sacrotuberous ligament
  - sacroiliac ligament (long dorsal, ventral and interosseous)
- the ligaments supporting the symphysis pubis joint including:
  - superior and inferior pubic ligaments
  - anterior and posterior pubic ligaments

- the ligaments supporting the lumbosacral joint:
  - iliolumbar ligament
  - thoracolumbar fascia

The active – muscle/fascia component of stability includes:
- the muscles stabilizing the sacroiliac joint including:
  - transverse abdominus via the thoracolumbar fascia
  - multifidus via the sacroiliac ligaments
  - piriformis
  - biceps femoris via the sacrotuberous ligament
  - pelvic muscle force field
  - gluteus maximus
- the muscles stabilizing the symphysis pubis joint including:
  - abdominals
  - pyramidalis
  - adductor longus which attaches across the joint
  - pelvic muscle force field
- the muscles stabilizing the lumbosacral joint including:
  - multifidus
  - erector spinae
  - quadratus lumborum via the lumbosacral ligament
  - abdominals via the thoracodorsal fascia
  - psoas

The control – neural component of stability includes:
- the autonomic nervous system
- the voluntary nervous system
- the integration of the two systems in muscle function

Analysis and description of the active – muscle/fascial component has focused on interaction of the abdominals and back musculature according to Lee. Only superficial attention has been paid to the pelvic floor and none to the PMFF. This book will begin the search and analysis of the PMFF's influence on the stability of the lumbo-pelvic region during physical activity.

The PMFF is composed of the pelvic diaphragm (levator ani), urogenital diaphragm, external sphincters, obturator internus, and adductor muscles. The PMFF facilitates lumbo-pelvic stability directly and indirectly:

1. Sapsford et. al. describes synergistic activity of the pelvic diaphragm (pubococcygeus) and the abdominals. When the pelvic diaphragm contracts the abdominals contract and vice versa. Thus when the PMFF acts it facilitates abdominal contraction which increases thoracodorsal fascia tension and intra-abdominal pressure to stabilize the lumbo-pelvic joints. In particular when the pubococcygeus contracts there is synergistic contraction of the transverse abdominus. The tranverse abdominus acts like a girdle squeezing around the lower abdomen and back, facilitating action of the multifidus and thoracolumbar fascia to support the lumbar spinal segments and lumbo-sacral junction. There is automatic stiffening of the spine and stabilizing of the pelvis.

2. Vleeming et. al. describes function of the dorsal and ventral sacroiliac ligaments in stabilizing the joint for back, arm, and leg movements. They prevent excessive sacral motion.
   a. Pelvic muscle force field - obturator phase - facilitates multifidus contraction.
   b. Pelvic muscle force field - abductor phase - facilitates transverse abdominus contraction.
   c. Together they facilitate ligamentous support of the sacroiliac joints in the neutral, stable position during functional activities.

3. Kapandji describes anterior symphysis pubis joint stability enhancement by the adductor longus muscle crossing over to attach on the pubic rami and blend with the anterior ligament. Bilateral adductor muscle contraction compresses the symphysis pubis joint and the anterior portion of the sacroiliac joints. At the same time it facilitates pelvic diaphragm contraction to counternutate the sacrum. This combination results in improved function of the sacroiliac region. The adductor longus and brevis force will be in the inferior direction rotating the pelvis anteriorly and counternutating the sacrum if the feet are planted. The adductor magnus, with its attachment to the ischial tuberosity may act to rotate the pelvis posteriorly. nutating the sacrum.

This further facilitates pelvic stability and balance.

4. The chain of fascia and ligaments from the foot to the lumbo-pelvic region is continuous such that distal movements of the lower leg and foot can assist in the stability of the pelvis. The pelvic diaphragm connects to the obturator internus at the arcuate tendon, which shares fibers with the sacrotuberous and sacrospinous ligaments, which interconnect with the biceps femoris, which attaches to the head of the fibula and the fascial connections of the peroneals, which attach on the navicular and the 5th metatarsal. Ankle and toe actions send a force through the interconnections to balance nutation and counternutaton of the sacrum for stability during gait and upper extremity activities.

5. The breathing diaphragm synergistically facilitates transverse abdominus action during the exhale phase of breathing. As the breathing diaphragm ascends, elevating the internal organs 1-3 cm and decreasing intra-abdominal pressures, the tranverse abdominus contracts, further stabilizing the lumbo-pelvic region.

Standing Balance

The ability to stand and balance is an amazing accompishment the result of many factors including musculoskeletal, motor control (neurologic), and sensory control. The musculoskeletal factors include hip stability and recovery from instability of postural sway movements. The presence of pain, alterations in joint range of motion, or alterations in muscle length or strength may produce dysfunction in balance. Muscle weakness, imbalance in muscle length or strength and/or lack of muscular endurance will effect balance. Motor control (neurologic) factors include components of the reflex model with higher levels of control utilizing the somatosensory, visual, and vestibular feedback loops. The brain integrates information ultimately determining the appropriate motor response from the sensory system. As sensory and motor systems change with age the speed of response decreases and the accuracy of the feedback loops decreases. The result is slower and less appropriate responses to outside perturbations in balance.

The PMFF is a key component in standing balance. It provides essential stability and force transfer through the pelvic and hip regions. Postural sway is, in part, movement of the pelvis around the lower extremities. Based on the ball and socket shape of the acetabulum and femoral head, any postural sway will have a significant rotational component. Since rotation is an integral part of both anterior and posterior sway and side-to-side sway, the PMFF with its rotation components facilitates subtle smooth responses to outside perturbations. The PMFF maintains sway within the midrange of motion over the base of support. It sets the stage from which the pelvis responds and the torso remains upright. It is the rotator cuff of the pelvis.

Ambulation

Each step is a PMFF action. The trunk participates in gait by rotating in a horizontal arc about the hip joint. This rotation will vary from subject to subject. The trunk winds and unwinds on the lower extremity with each walking cycle. From heel strike to toe off, the pelvis rotates clockwise and the femur rotates medially. Beginning with toe off and during swing phase the pelvis rotates counterclockwise and the femur rotates laterally. After heel strike the weight is transferred along the lateral border of the foot with foot inversion. The weight is then transferred across the transverse arch to the big toe for push off with simultaneous hip medial rotation and ankle eversion. The PMFF is continually active during all phases of ambulation to accomplish the small amplitudes of midrange rotation. According to Inman et. al. pelvic rotation is one of the major determinants of locomotion that serves to lessen the amplitude of the vertical excursion of the center of gravity of the body during each step, thus decreasing energy expenditure of gait. Pelvic rotation also appears to be a means of elongating the step length when walking conditions require it. When hip rotation is limited gait is significantly impacted. Hip rotation decreases with age from a mean of 50° each direction at nine years of age to 22° medial and 32° lateral rotation at 65 years of age. Pelvic rotation and step length both decrease with age.

The medial and lateral hip rotator muscles are active in gait. These two groups work together throughout gait to improve efficiency, maintain balance, and assist in transfer of force from the outside to the inside of the foot over even or uneven terrain. The lateral rotator group includes the obturator internus and externus, the superior and inferior gemelli, the quadratus femoris, and the piriformis muscles. The medial rotator group includes the adductors, gracilis, pectineus, and to some extent gluteus minimus and medius muscles. If for any reason there is an imbalance in function between these two groups gait will be altered and balance will be compromised. For example, if there is shortening or spasm of trigger points in the adductors of the medial rotator group the resulting reflex inhibition of the lateral rotators will significantly alter movement above and below this axis. Pelvic and trunk rotation in the horizontal plane will be altered as well as the significant rotary components at the ankle, foot and knee that enable transfer of weight from heel to big toe for push off. When the adductors dominate action over the outward rotators the base of support narrows during dual stance. In an extreme case the feet cross over one another. The PMFF assists in effective stability during the stance phase and efficient mobility during the swing phase of gait. Thus the PMFF functions as the dynamic rotator cuff of the pelvis.

Chapter 10

Neurology of Chronic Pelvic Pain and Low Back Pain

Neurology of Continence

The **voluntary nervous system,** from **sacral nerve roots 2, 3 & 4** senses and receives information from the pelvic and urogenital diaphragm and external sphincter muscles via the **pudendal nerve.** The voluntary nervous system, from sacral nerve roots 2, 3 & 4 via the **pelvic nerve** innervates the obturator internus.

The **autonomic nervous system** innervates the bladder, urethra, bowel and rectum. There are three divisions of the autonomic nervous system:

the **sympathetic system** (fight or flight system)
hypogastric plexus - nerve roots **thoracic 10, 11, 12, lumbar 1 & 2** innervates primarily bladder neck and proximal urethra.

the **parasympathetic system**
pelvic plexus - nerve roots **sacral 2, 3 & 4** innervates primarily the bladder wall

the **enteric system** gastrointestinal nerve plexus. (Figure 9)

AUTONOMIC NERVOUS SYSTEM		
Parasympathetic	Enteric	Sympathetic
craniosacral nerve roots	gastrointestinal nerve plexus	thoracolumbar nerve roots

Figure 9

The voluntary and autonomic nervous system work together to maintain continence. (Figure 10) For 24 hours of the day the pelvic diaphragm maintains a resting tone adequate to position the bladder and assist in closure of the bladder neck/proximal urethra (a striated muscle's resting tone is largely determined by the ANS). At the same time the detrusor muscle is maintaining a resting level adequate to allow expansion of bladder size without setting off muscle contractions (largely through inhibition of smooth muscle contraction by the ANS).

When the urge to urinate or have a bowel movement is perceived in the brain the voluntary nervous system comes into play stimulating the pelvic diaphragm and external sphincters to contract volitionally. The spinal reflex arc causes the detrusor muscle contractions to be inhibited.

This implies that afferent messages from the voluntary nervous

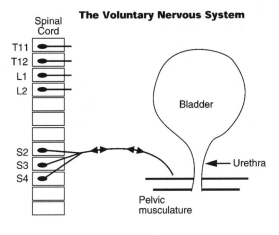

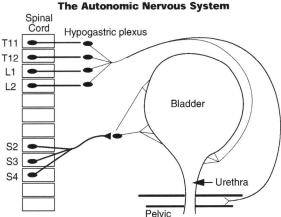

Figure 10 The Nervous System

system travel to the spinal cord synapse with autonomic efferent fibers to transmit inhibitory messages to the bladder wall.

As many as sixteen reflex arcs exist between the bowel, bladder, spinal cord and brain, all of which control continence.

From birth to approximately three years of age elimination is controlled primarily by the pons. At approximately three, when a child can begin to count and say the A•B•Cs, the cortex becomes dominant in elimination control and potty training is successful. Until this point the caretaker is trained more so than the child. In the elderly, as cognitive function declines, the pons again becomes the more dominant force in elimination. Pons control is an unconscious process – when the afferent messages of bladder stretching are received the efferent message is to pause, release the pelvic muscles and eliminate the urine or feces without concern for time or place.

The **enteric nervous** system is the third division of the autonomic nervous system. It is known as the "gut's" brain. Located in tissue lining the esophagus, stomach, small intestine and colon, it is a complex neural network of electrical and chemical messengers that can function in isolation from the central nervous system. This complex of integrated circuits, blood brain barriers, and chemical and hormone production centers, acts interdependently with the central nervous system via the vagus nerve. The vagus nerve consists of 2000 parasympathetic nerve fibers innervating the heart and gut. There is dual innervation of the throat, and upper two-thirds of the stomach, rectum and anus. The small intestine and large intestine are innervated by only the enteric nervous system. The small intestine contains 100 million enteric neurons, somewhat surprisingly more than exist in the spinal cord. The enteric system produces the same neurotransmitters found in the brain, including serotonin, dopamine, norepinephrine, nitric oxide, enkephalins, benzodiazapines, neuropeptides, and immune system cells. It produces 95% of the body's serotonin. The gut brain effects the head brain as much or more so than vice versa. Much of abdominal and pelvic pain, difficulty swallowing, bowel problems and to some extent bladder problems originate from gut brain-enteric nervous system dysfunction. Treating the enteric nervous system is essential to improving CPP.

Pain Perception

Pain travels via both somatic and visceral afferent nerves, sensory nerves. (Figure 11) Somatic afferent nerves transmit information from skin, subcutaneous tissue, skeletal muscle, and parietal peritoneum. When there are trigger points in muscle, pain can be referred through somatic afferent nerves from the muscle to the motor/sensory area of the brain via the dorsal horn of the spinal cord. The pain felt is sharp and localized. Visceral afferent nerves transmit information from abdominal and pelvic viscera, sweat glands, organs, visceral peritoneum, and blood vessels. When there is pain producing sensations in these structures it is transmitted to the dorsal horn of the spinal cord and then to both the limbic (emotional) system and prefrontal cortex of the brain. This pain is felt in a general area and described with an emotional component as terrible or dreadful.

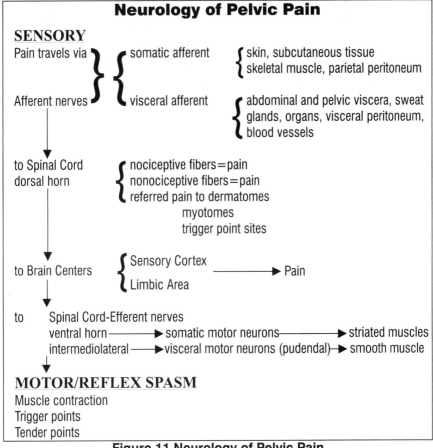

Figure 11 Neurology of Pelvic Pain

Pain travels through sensory nociceptive nerve fibers that are unmyelinated or poorly myelinated. In the dorsal horn of the spinal cord the visceral nociceptor fibers influence somatic sensory and somatic motor fibers via interneurons. The somatic sensory and motor fibers can be sensitized by the visceral nociceptor fibers of the same proximal spinal cord level. This is called **viscerosomatic convergence**.

The lack of insulation, allows irritation or stimulation of many other nerve fibers at the dorsal horn level of the spinal cord. Fifteen to twenty additional fibers may be stimulated or irritated by one visceral

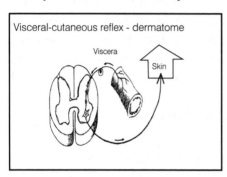
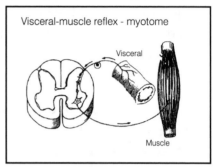

Figure 12 Visceral cutaneous & visceral muscle reflexes

nociceptive nerve. This is called **crosstalk.**

Viscerosomatic convergence and crosstalk enable visceral pain to be referred to striated muscle in the form of turgor or spasm in the same or related **myotome** spinal segment. Individuals describe muscle spasm in specific abdominal, groin, back and buttocks myotomal patterns. (Figure 12)

Viscerosomatic convergence and crosstalk explain visceral pain that is localized to skin and subcutaneous tissue of the same or related **dermatome** spinal segment. (Figure 12) Individuals describe pain in specific abdominal, groin, back and buttocks dermatomal patterns. (Figure 13)

Descending messages from the limbic system of the brain influence pain through interneuron connections to somatic and visceral afferents in the dorsal horn of the spinal cord. The limbic system or hypothalamus-pituitary-adrenal (HPA) axis, is known as the stress axis of the body. The response of the limbic system to fatigue, trauma, emotional, psychological, or anticipatory stressors is to increase the stress chemicals/hormones produced. An increase in cortisol, epinephrine,

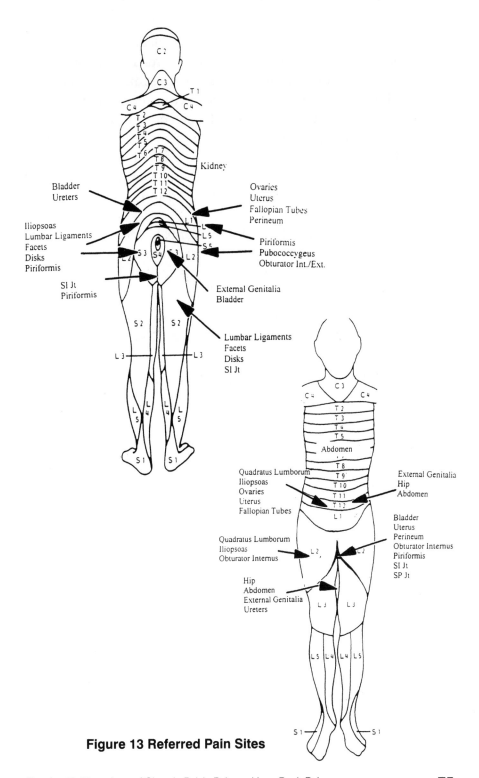

Figure 13 Referred Pain Sites

and substance P effects every cell of the body including the interneuron connections in the dorsal horn of the spinal cord. The limbic system influences the autonomic nervous system leading to increased sympathetic drive. Increased sympathetic drive increases muscle resting tone and decreases circulation to muscles and other tissues.

Ischemia of muscles or nerves results in chemical changes including increased lactic acid, potassium, histamine, and bradykinin. Following any tissue damage or inflammation there are increased levels of prostaglandins. These chemical changes lead to extreme tenderness and pain.

Another influence in CPP is the level of pain enhancing and pain modulating chemicals present in the dorsal horn of the spinal cord. (Figure 14) Non-nociceptive sensory fibers for touch, pressure, and temperature typically have opiate influence as they connect with

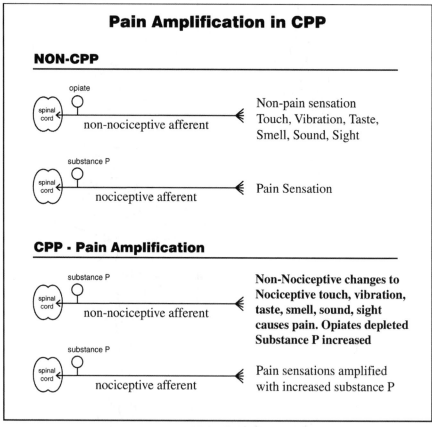

Figure 14 Pain Amplification

interneurons in the spinal cord. The opiate receptors are stimulated by serotonin, which modulates any pain perception. If serotonin is depleted, the influence of substance P on the non-nociceptive sensory fibers increases. Substance P is a pain enhancer, so with chronic pain substance P can become a predominant influence. Non-nociceptive fibers can become nociceptive in nature. In other words, touch, pressure or temperature change is perceived in the brain as pain. In addition, the nociceptive pain fibers primary neurotransmitter is substance P. Extreme response to pain is modulated in nociceptive fibers by opiods/enkephalins, so depletion of opiods or their precursor serotonin, results in increased pain perception via nociceptive fiber transmissions. The same opiod and substance P influence is present in the limbic system of the brain.

Chronic pelvic pain may originate with a minor injury or dysfunction that long ago has been resolved. The chronic response of the nervous systems and brain have since resulted in long term imbalance of the sympathetic-parasympathetic drive, chronic activation of the limbic system (HPA axis), overabundance of substance P, lack of opiates, and ischemia to muscles and nerves from constricted blood vessels. The result is increased muscle resting tone and an inability of muscle to rest even during sleep, disrupted sleep patterns and disrupted breathing patterns. The brain perceives this long term disruption in homeostasis as pain and fatigue.

Neural Control of Lumbo-Pelvic Stability

Muscle control of lumbo-pelvic stability is effected by the neurology of lumbo-pelvic joints, which is significantly effected by the neurology of the muscular system surrounding the lumbo-pelvic area. Spinal segments lumbar 5, sacral 1, 2, 3 & 4 provide both autonomic and voluntary nervous system nerve roots which innervate the joint structures and the muscles of the lumbo-pelvic area. According to Wyke mechanoreceptors of the joints and the muscles (muscle spindle) effect movement and stability through automatic reflex responses, postural and kinesthetic responses and pain responses. These mechanoreceptors have reflexogenic effects on muscle resting tone and the excitability of the stretch reflex in muscle action. They also have significant input to reflex inhibition of opposing muscles resulting in smooth, graded movement in joint structures. When dysfunction or injury to joints or muscles occurs, or their innervation or circulation is interrupted, the stability of the lumbo-pelvic region is compromised.

Any disruption in the neurology of the system results in changes throughout the system. Visualize a small pebble thrown into a pond with the resulting waves spreading to the far reaches of the pond's surface. Likewise, a small constriction of blood to the pelvic nerve innervating the obturator internus muscle will impact the entire PMFF, the internal organs of bladder, bowel, uterus, in addition to the sacroiliac joint, symphysis pubis joint and low back.

The autonomic nervous system response to a small pebble in the pond is to send a system wide alarm, the intensity of which is determined by how dangerous the CNS perceives the danger. The goal of the ANS is to wall off the area saving the rest of the body, and then to repair the local area through protection and regeneration.

When it is understood that preservation of the rest of the body is paramount it is easier to understand why the circulation is decreased to the injured site, the muscles tighten around the site, and the nervous system sends vital nutrition to organs, brain, and other tissues to keep them functioning. Over the long term the local site often heals but the muscles and circulation surrounding the site continue to function in a pattern similar to the emergency edict. Circulation continues to be impaired, muscles continue to be abnormally tight during rest and they are uncoordinated during movement. The result is pain, postural changes, and abnormal body movement directed to a large extent by the ans. The fight or flight system, the sympathetic division, is on high drive compared to the parasympathetic, quieting system. In general, sleep is disrupted, total movement patterns are inefficient, and fatigue is a major complaint. More locally, circulation is decreased to muscles, tendons, joints, and nerves. Muscles have high resting tone controlled by the sympathetic input to the muscle spindle. There is accumulation of waste products in the tissues and decreased oxygen and food product transport to the muscle cells. Joints become excessively compressed.

Physics teaches us that for every action there is an equal and opposite reaction. In the body this equal and opposite reaction includes an overactive reflex inhibition of opposing muscles, increased joint laxity underlying these muscles, and depressed stretch reflexes above, below, or on the opposite side of the injury. Over the long term when the affected anatomy is located in the lower abdomen, back or pelvis, these dysfunctions lead to chronic low back and/or pelvic pain.

The goal of a program to improve neural control of lumbo-pelvic stability is to regain the balance between sympathetic and parasympathetic input to the associated structures and should lead to normal and efficient rest patterns. The ANS controls circulation, muscle resting tone, and oxygen/food transport. An effective program to balance the ANS is Physiological Quieting.

What are Trigger Points and Tender Points?

Trigger points are hypersensitive spots in skeletal muscle associated with palpable nodules in taut bands. Trigger points refer pain, tenderness, spasm and autonomic changes to areas distal from the original point of tenderness. The point is tender and the taut band prevents the muscle from stretching to its full length. Trigger points decrease functional strength of muscle. Pressure or stretch results in a contraction of the effected muscles. A primary trigger point can activate more peripheral secondary points.

It is thought that trigger points are caused by dysfunction at the neuromuscular junction. Evaluated with electromyography, they appear as spontaneous electrical activity and the referred symptoms are mediated through interneuron connections at the spinal cord level. The tight bands in the muscle may be microscopic contraction within the endplates of the muscle fibers. Trigger points are characteristic of myofascial pain syndrome diagnosis.

Tender points are hypersensitive spots in skeletal muscle that do not refer pain or tenderness from the original point of tenderness. In both trigger points and tender points 3-5 kg of pressure elicit acute symptoms. Tender points are characteristic of a fibromyalgia diagnosis.

Perpetuating factors for trigger points and tender points include enzyme dysfunctions that interfere with muscle energy metabolism. Vitamin deficiencies that contribute to enzyme deficiencies include C, B1, B6, B12, and folic acid. Low levels of potassium, calcium, magnesium, and trace minerals also contribute to trigger points and tender point severity.

Hypoestrogenism (low estrogen levels), hypothyroidism, anemia, and hypoglycemia aggravate trigger point and tender point symptoms. Any myofascial therapy will be ineffective until these nutritional problems are addressed.

Postural dysfunction, repetitive motion at home or work, positional stretch or compression can be perpetuating factors as well. Asymmetrical postures, scoliosis, leg length discrepancy, and foot deformity can perpetuate the pain and tenderness of trigger points. Excessive repetitive work patterns without balanced rest cycles stimulate trigger point symptoms. Extended periods in a stretched or shortened position without movement, for example during sleep or surgery, can also elicit symptoms of trigger points.

The components of chronic pelvic pain assessment include:
  History
  Special Questions
  Daily Diary
  Functional Impact Questionnaire
  Physical Assessment
  Neuromuscular Assessment (Biofeedback)

Chapter 11

History and Special Questions

History

What are the questions to ask?

In taking the history, both general and specific questions will provide the basis for an appropriate physical examination and differential diagnosis. General questions include pain pattern characteristics, pain pattern perception, involvement of associated organ functions, daily functional alterations, medications, emotional aspects, and desired goals. Initially the individual completes the CPP and LBP Questionnaire Packet. (page 90)

Chronic Pelvic Pain History Form

I. Present Symptoms
   A. Symptom Picture
      1. Draw a picture (Figure 15)
      2. Location (Figure 16)
   B. Symptom Pattern
      1. Frequency of symptoms
      2. Daily and nightly patterns
   C. Symptom Intensity
      1. Pain algorithm 0-10 scale 0= no pain, 10= extreme pain
      2. Do you feel you have high or low pain tolerance?
      3. What is the intensity during the last month, week, day?
   D. Pain Description
      1. Sharp, dull, throbbing, shooting, cramping, colicky
   E. Symptoms' Affect on Function (Figure 17, 18, 19)
      1. Work, home, social, recreational activities?
      2. Describe your lifestyle before the onset of CPP.
      3. Is it easy or hard to have fun?
      4. Do daily activities increase symptoms? How?

II. Symptom History
   A. Type of onset
   B. Duration since onset
   C. Pattern since onset
   D. Treatments tried – medication, surgical, counseling, etc.

III. Bladder Symptoms (Figure 20)
   A. Frequency, urgency day/night
   B. Discomfort with urination/ relief of pain with urination
   C. Flow strength, ease of starting and stopping
   D. Urine color, odor, blood
   E. Uncontrolled loss of urine
   F. Urinary tract infection frequency
   G. Perception of complete emptying

IV. Bowel Symptoms (Figure 20)
   A. Frequency of elimination
   B. Consistency and appearance of stool

    C. Strain or urgency to eliminate

    D. Change in bowel habits

    E. Pain, discomfort or relief of pain with elimination

    F. Anal discharge, leaking, uncontrolled loss of feces

    G. Incomplete emptying

    H. Bloating, distension, flatulence

V. Associated Symptoms (Figure 16)

    A. Breathing pattern- shortness of breath, breath holding

    B. Headaches, neck pain

    C. Cold hands and/or feet

    D. Premenstrual syndrome (PMS) symptoms

    E. Sexual function- orgasm, libido

    F. Depression, anxiety symptoms

    G. Post traumatic stress disorder (PTSD)

        1. physical, emotional, sexual abuse

VI. Sleep/Wake Patterns (Figure 21)

    A. Time to get to sleep

    B. Frequency of awakenings

    C. Perception of restfulness in the morning

    D. Regular bed and awaken times

    E. Total hours sleep/night

VII. Other Medical Problems

    A. Infections- yeast, vaginal, bladder

    B. Allergies

    C. Surgeries- hysterectomy, back, abdominal, pelvic, brain, laparoscopy

    D. Radiation, chemotherapy

VIII. Reproductive History

    A. Menstruation

        1. Age of initiation

        2. Symptoms

        3. Length and regularity

    B. Pregnancy

        1. Number of pregnancies, number of live births

        2. Number of cesareans, miscarriages, abortions

Special Questions

There are specific questions that can be asked during the history portion of assessment that can lead to more specific tests and a more accurate diagnosis. The diagnosis and specific questions include:

Adhesions

1. Is there a history of pelvic surgery, pelvic inflammatory disease, irritable bowel syndrome, endometriosis, or deep dyspareunia?
2. Does the pain vary with movement or activity?
3. Is the pain sharp and intermittent?
4. Does the pain vary with the menstrual cycle?

Pain can originate in the parietal peritoneum and the adhesions themselves as both have been found to contain nerve fibers. The pain tends to increase with movement and be more sharp and intermittent than dull and constant. The pain may vary with the menstrual cycle and deep dyspareunia is often present.

Dysmenorrhea

1. Is the pain associated with menstruation?
2. Are there PMS symptoms before or during menstruation?
3. Is there a history of sexually transmitted disease (STDs)?

Dysmenorrhea is described by individuals as severe, cramping pain in the lower abdomen, low back and upper thighs during or just before menses. There is primary and secondary dysmenorrhea. Primary dysmenorrhea is present when there is no pelvic pathology. Secondary dysmenorrhea is present when there is pelvic pathology that is the cause of the pain, i.e. STDs. A widely accepted theory of the cause of primary dysmenorrhea is that there is an abnormal increase in prostaglandin levels that stimulates excessive, abnormal uterine contractions. Vasopressin, a powerful uterine muscle stimulant, increases fourfold during menstruation and may be a factor in dysmenorrhea.

Dyspareunia

1. Is there pain with intercourse?
2. Is the pain experienced before, at entry, during, with deep thrusting, or after?
3. What type of pain do you experience?

Causes of dyspareunia can include anal fissures, duct obstructions, hypoestrogenation, endometriosis, adhesions, ovarian or uterine pathology or malposition, or pelvic muscle dysfunction.

Endometriosis

1. Did the pain begin as menstrual cramps?
2. Is the pain worse just before or with menses?
3. Is there pain with deep penetration during intercourse? Does it continue afterward?
4. Is there rectal pain, especially with bowel movements?
5. Are there problems conceiving?
6. Is there irregular uterine bleeding, particularly between-period bleeding?

Endometriosis is the presence of endometrium located outside the endometrial cavity of the uterus. It has been found on ovaries, ligaments, appendix, peritoneum, bladder, lymph nodes, vagina, cervix, and fallopian tubes to name a few. The pain often appears initially as dysmenorrhea, being worse the first 2 or 3 days of the menstrual cycle and may be present several days before menstruation begins. Pain with intercourse is common. Rectal pain often indicates involvement of the uterosacral ligament, rectum or vaginal areas. Between period bleeding is a common complaint.

Pelvic Varicosities/ Pelvic Congestion Syndrome

1. Is there pain on one side or both sides? Is there low back pain?
2. Is the pain dull and aching?
3. Is the pain increased by movement or walking?
4. Is the pain more severe premenstrually?
5. Is there pain with intercourse or after?
6. Are headaches, fatigue, or insomnia present?
7. Is there irregular or heavy menstrual bleeding or between-period bleeding?

In this condition pelvic veins are dilated and the valves are poorly functioning leading to pelvic vein varicosities, much like varicosities in the legs. Symptoms include dull, aching pelvic pain with acute periods of sharp pain, sacral pain, and deep dyspareunia. Pain often increases before and during menstruation.

Neurally Mediated Hypotension

1. Is there low blood pressure and/or high resting heart rate?
2. Do symptoms include feeling dizzy and weak in the knees when arising from supine?
3. Is pain more severe premenstrually?
4. Is pain relieved by lying down compared to being upright?
5. Are there problems with indigestion, swallowing and bowel movements?

In this condition the individual experiences chronic low blood pressure and often high resting heart rate. Heart rate can be 90-100 beats/min. at rest. Blood pressure can be 90/65 mm Hg or lower. Symptoms include mental and physical fatigue, chest and abdominal pain, swallowing and indigestion problems.

Reproductive Hormonal Deregulation

1. Are there monthly cycles of abdominal and pelvic pain?
2. Are there yearly cycles of increased abdominal/pelvic pain?
3. Are there menstrual irregularities?
4. Are there monthly cycles of bladder and bowel irritability?

In this condition the individual often experiences cyclic increased muscle pain, fatigue, sleep disturbance, menstrual irregularities, bowel and bladder irritability and depression.

Pelvic Floor Relaxation Syndromes

1. Are there feelings of pressure, heaviness, aching, and a falling out feeling in the lower pelvis when standing for any length of time?
2. Do symptoms include loss of urine with cough, constipation, pelvic pain, and urinary urgency?
3. Is there a history of vaginal delivery, extended length of second stage labor, large baby, complications, tears or episiotomies?
4. Is there pain or lack of feeling with intercourse?

In this condition individuals experience pressure, heaviness, a "falling out" feeling, and back ache with standing. Uncontrolled loss of urine and constipation may be present. Inability to empty the bladder or bowel can be experienced. There may be pain during intercourse.

Vulvodynia/Vulvar Vestibulitis

1. Are there symptoms including vulvar hypersensitivity, itching, burning, vaginal pain, and dyspareunia?
2. Is pain aggravated by perspiration, semen, tight clothing, or sitting?
3. Is there pelvic aching after intercourse?
4. Is there a history of bacterial infections, diabetes, vulvar surgery or trauma?

In this condition individuals describe burning, stinging, irritation, and rawness in the area of the female external genitalia, and dyspareunia during intercourse.

Interstitial Cystitis (IC)

1. Is there urinary frequency day and night?
2. Is there uncontrolled loss of urine?
3. Is there pain or discomfort with urination?
4. Is there pain with a full bladder and relief after emptying the bladder?
5. Is there a childhood history of infections, leaking or bed-wetting?

Unremitting frequency, urgency and nocturia are the primary symptoms of IC. Fifty to seventy percent of individuals with IC complain of pelvic pain, usually located suprapubically. It may radiate into the back and groin. Most women with IC also experience dyspareunia. In many individuals pain increases with bladder filling and decreases after voiding. Pain with urinating is occasionally present.

Nerve Entrapment

1. Is the onset of pain related to recent or past trauma or surgery in the pain region?
2. Is there any increase or decrease in sensitivity of the skin in the pain region?
3. Is the pain sharp, shooting and intermittent?

In this condition the individual can experience hyperesthesia, sensory loss, tenderness, and motor loss in the distribution of the specific nerve.

Hypoglycemia/Reactive Hypoglycemia Tendencies

1. Are there symptoms including shakiness, weakness, pain and fatigue, irritability/irrationality soon after a meal?
2. Is there a craving for sweets or fat and protein?
3. Are blood glucose levels below 95 mg/dl?

In this condition the individual can experience shakiness, weakness, pain and fatigue, irritability and irrationality. If it occurs within 30-40 minutes after a meal it is called reactive hypoglycemia and is relieved by eating fat and protein. If symptoms occur 1-2 hours after a meal it is called general hypoglycemia and eating carbohydrates relieves the symptoms.

Hypothyroid Tendencies

1. Are there symptoms of fatigue, pain, dry skin, heavy periods, hair loss, weight gain and constipation?
2. Are there complaints of cold hands and feet – of being core cold?
3. Is basal body temperature at or below 97.6°?

In this condition the individual can experience symptoms of fatigue and pain in addition to hair loss, dry skin, constipation and weight gain. Blood tests will be normal. Basal body temperature testing will indicate that T4 to T3 conversion at the cellular level is potentially deficient.

Post Traumatic Stress Disorder

1. Are there symptoms of sadness and/or tears most days?
2. Is there a significant loss of interest or pleasure in usual activities?
3. Is there significant weight change?
4. Have sleep patterns changed, i.e. can't sleep or sleep all the time?
5. Is there a lack of energy or fatigue daily?
6. Are there problems making decisions, thinking, or concentrating?
7. Are there significant changes in social, occupational or personal life style?
8. Is there a history of depression, chemical or drug dependency?

In this condition the individual can experience sadness and tears, with a loss of interest or pleasure in daily activities. Fatigue is present. Sleep is often disrupted. Some individuals sleep excessively. Concentration, decision making and learning is compromised. There is often a history of depression, chemical or drug dependency.

Chronic Pelvic Pain and Low Back Pain

Questionaire Packet

Complete the following questionaires and bring them to the first clinic visit.

_____   _____
Name   Date

Draw the location of your pain

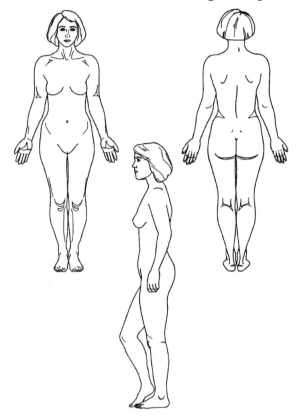

Pain Level (0=no pain   10=excruciating pain)

0   1   2   3   4   5   6   7   8   9   10

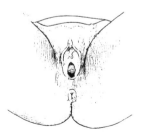

Pain Level (0=no pain   10=excruciating pain)

0   1   2   3   4   5   6   7   8   9   10

Figure 15 Pain Patterns

CPP & LBP Questionaire

Check the appropriate boxes that describe you in the last two weeks.

General Characteristics

Yes	Pain	Location	Right	Left
	Abdomen			
	Back			
	Buttocks			
	Legs			
	Vagina			
	Anus			
	Other			

Yes	Fatigue
	Mental
	Physical
	Other

Yes	Sleep Disturbance
	Unable to get to sleep in <30 min.
	Multiple awakenings a night
	Awaken feeling tired

Yes	Daily Activity disturbance	
	Self care	List:
	Work	List
	Social/Recreational	List:

Associated Symptoms

Yes	Symptom
	Headaches
	Memory Problems
	Allergies

Yes	Symptom
	Cold Hands or Feet
	Bowel Irregularities
	Bladder Irregularities

	Dry Mouth
	Blurred Vision
	Neck Pain/Upper Back Pain
	Jaw Pain

	Restless Leg Syndrome
	Hearing Irregularities
	Heart Palpitations
	Shortness of Breath

	Stiffness
	Numbness/Tingling
	Swelling
	Clumsiness

	Anxiety
	Depression
	Sexual Dysfunction
	Other

Figure 16

Symptom Pattern and Variation Questionairre

Describe:

When do I feel.....	the Best	the Worst	Symptoms
Days of the Month			
Days of the Week			
Times of the Day			
Activities			

Foods/Nutrients			
Other			

When I feel lousy what helps the symptoms?

_____

_____

Figure 17

Work / Rest Cycle Report

Record the minutes of work time you can perform without increasing pain and fatigue. Then report the minutes of rest time needed between work cycles to keep pain at a minimum.

minutes **Work** activity	**Rest**
1.	
2.	
3.	

Figure 18

Chronic Pelvic Pain Functional Impact Questionnaire

Rate your overall quality of life.

   0   1   2   3   4   5   6   7   8   9   10
   Very Poor   Excellent
   (As bad as it can get)   (As good as it can get)

Rate how much your pain interferes with each of the following:

1. Self care – dressing, bathing, hair care.

   0   1   2   3   4   5   6   7   8   9   10
   Does not Interfere   Completely Interferes

2. Daily activities – cooking, cleaning, laundry, shopping, hobbies.

   0   1   2   3   4   5   6   7   8   9   10
   Does not Interfere   Completely Interferes

3. Ability to work outisde the home or go to school.

   0   1   2   3   4   5   6   7   8   9   10
   Does not Interfere   Completely Interferes

4. Social interaction: visiting friends, social activities in or out of home, volunteer activities.

   0   1   2   3   4   5   6   7   8   9   10
   Does not Interfere   Completely Interferes

5. Sleep: adequate sleep, feeling rested when awaken.

   0   1   2   3   4   5   6   7   8   9   10
   Does not Interfere   Completely Interferes

6. Sexual relationships.

   0   1   2   3   4   5   6   7   8   9   10
   Does not Interfere   Completely Interferes

7. Ability to enjoy life.

   0   1   2   3   4   5   6   7   8   9   10
   Does not Interfere   Completely Interferes

8. Self perception: physical health, mental health.

   0   1   2   3   4   5   6   7   8   9   10
   Does not Interfere   Completely Interferes

(With Permission – Penner. B.)

Figure 19 CPP Functional Impact Questionnaire

Bladder-Bowel Diary

Name_____

Week of_____

Instructions

Insert the following symbols into the appropriate time spaces

T = toilet
B = bowel movement
F = 8oz. fluid
* = caffeinated
L = small leak
A = large leak
P = pad

Day____Date_____
6-8 am
8-10
10-12
12-2 pm
2-4
4-6
6-8
8-10
10-12
Overnight
Pads used (comments)

Day____Date_____
6-8 am
8-10
10-12
12-2 pm
2-4
4-6
6-8
8-10
10-12
Overnight
Pads used (comments)

Day____Date_____
6-8 am
8-10
10-12
12-2 pm
2-4
4-6
6-8
8-10
10-12
Overnight
Pads used (comments)

Figure 20 Daily Diary

Weekly Self-Care Report

Report your symptoms and activities according to the following guidelines.

Rate your pain on a 0-10 scale. 0 = no pain   10 = excruciating pain

Indicate activities and rest periods.   R=Rest
                                           E=Exercise
                                           W=Work
                                           P=Play

Indicate hours slept and number of awakenings in the parenthesis ( ). See the following example.

Date: _3/21/01_

_4 W_ _____ _8_ ____ _E R 6 W_ ____ _10_ _____ (_6_ / _6_)

awaken   lunch   dinner   bedtime

Comments: _____

_____

Date:_____

_____ (/   )

awaken   lunch   dinner   bedtime

Comments: _____

_____

_____

Date:_____

_____ (/   )

awaken   lunch   dinner   bedtime

Comments: _____

_____

_____

Date:_____

_____ (/   )

awaken   lunch   dinner   bedtime

Comments: _____

_____

Figure 21

Chapter 12

Physical Assessment

Observe Affective Domain

Movement Patterns: walking, sit to stand, bending
Facial Expressions
Overall Appearance: dress, hair, make-up

Basic Physiological Tests

Blood pressure   Blood Glucose levels
Heart Rate   Basal Body Temperature

Standing Assessment   Observe For:

Posture   Alignment of:

Front: Shoulders, umbilicus, linea alba, iliac crest, ASIS, patella, medial malleolus
Back: Shoulders, scapula, spine, iliac crests, SI, knees, medial malleolus
Side: Mastoid process, shoulder, hip, knee, ankle

Motion
Forward bend	Typical pelvic pain posture
Sidebend	Scoliosis
Rotation	Range of motion limits

One Leg Standing	Laxity of the pubic symphysis
With hip flexion	Laxity of pelvic girdle
	Weakness of hip and pelvis
Iliac Crest Symmetry	Short leg syndrome

March Test	Sacroiliac joint dysfunction
Cruising	Hip rotator muscle dysfunction
Plie	Hip and pelvic muscle synergy deficit
Gait	Short leg syndrome
	Herniated disc
	General musculoskeletal problems
Fibromyalgia Test	Tender points

Sitting Assessment

Posture – Observe	Back – general tone, paraspinal symmetry
	Lower trapezius symmetry, scoliosis
	Inferior angle of scapula
	Abdomen – muscle symmetry, linea alba integrity
	Skin color, texture, hair, defects
Sensory Testing	Visceral referral pain
sharp, dull, light touch	Herniated disc
Palpation	
Upper and Lower Back	Trigger points
	Myalgia
Iliac Crests	Symmetry
	Trigger points
Sacrum	Trigger points
	Sacroilitis
Leg Length	Leg length discrepancy
Long sitting	
Muscle Strength Test	Herniated disc
	Sacral roots 2-4

Prone Assessment

Alignment	Lumbar and hip position
Observe Condition low back, sacrum, gluteal, lower extremities	Swelling, edema Symmetry
Legs straight Knees flexed	Anterior/posterior tilt

Palpation and accessory motion

Iliac crests	Sacral tilt
Sacral base	Sacral torsion
Sacral angle	
Lumbar facets	Facet syndrome
Sacroiliac joints	Hyper/hypomobility

Palpation	Trigger points
Gluteals	Spasm
Piriformis	
Hamstrings	
Erector Spinae	
Quadratus Lumborum	

Supine Assessment

Observe Condition

Abdomen/Groin	Abdominal swelling, distension
Valsalva, cough	Femoral, inguinal bulges
	Scars, muscle asymmetry
Lower Extremities	Symmetry, swelling, edema, scars
Pelvic Posture	Lumbar and hip position
	Tilt- anterior/posterior

Abdominal/Groin

Sensation
    Gentle Pinching   Referred visceral pain
    Basic Sensory Test   Neuropathy
    Light, dull   Nerve entrapment

Abdominal/Groin   Trigger points
Palpation   Myofascial pain
                            Nerve entrapment
                            Incisional scar entrapment
                            Hernias
                            Ovarian point tenderness
                            Inguinal ring
                            Tenderness, guarding, masses

Muscle Length Tests   see Figure 22

Muscle Strength Tests   see Figure 22
Head Raise, Leg Raise   Linea alba separation
                            Abdominal muscle weakness
                            Disc herniation
                            Low back dysfunction
Knee to chest   Low back pain
                            Abdominal muscle weakness
                            Deconditioning
Obturator and Psoas   Shortening, dysfunction, spasm
    Sign Tests

Hip Clearing Test   Hip pathology

Sacroiliac Compression   Sacroiliac dysfunction
    Distraction

Pubic Symphysis   Trigger points
    palpation   Accessory motion limits
    accessory motion   Pain

Urogenital and Pelvic Muscle Force Field (PMFF) Assessment

Observe Labia and External Genitalia	Inflammation, abscesses, ulcerations Color changes, exudates, fissures, atrophy
Basic Sensory Tests Sharp, dull, light touch	Nerve entrapment Neuropathy Spinal cord lesion
Vestibule Test w/ cotton swab	Vulvar vestibulitis pain
Anal Wink Test	Reflex innervation High tone, decr wink
Single Digit Palpation Vulva, Pubic Arch Introitus/ Bulbospon Levator Ani Arcuate Tendon Coccygeus Obturator Internus Piriformis Urethra and Trigone area	see Figure 23 Trigger points Vaginisimus, trigger points Resting tone Urethral Syndrome Urethritis Cystitis, Trigonitis Interstitial Cystitis
Rectum	Irritable Bowel Syndrome / Tone
Observation With Valsalva	Enterocele Rectocele Cystocele Uterine Prolapse

Neuromuscular Assessment with Biofeedback

PMFF Functional Tests (with vaginal/anal/surface EMG) (Fig. 24)

Resting	Resting tone
Quick Contraction	Type II fiber function, Urogenital diaphragm
Ten Second Hold	Type I fiber function,
Isolated	Pelvic diaphragm
Obturator Assist	Obturator internus
Adductor Assist	Adductors
Release	Return to rest function
Valsalva	Reflex support
Standing Plie	PMFF functional position

Note: Report on amplitude, duration, latency to peak and latency in return to rest of monitored muscles. Report accessory muscles used. Report resting level characteristics. Compare amplitude and duration of three types of 10 second holds.

Stress Tests (with surface EMG, thermal, and respiration) (Fig. 25)

Baseline	Resting tone
Math	ANS- muscle spindle
Stress Story	ANS- blood vessel
Pain Story	ANS- diaphragm/respiration
Rest Return	Return to rest level

Mobility Tests

Baseline	Resting tone
Flexion	Muscle symmetry
Rotation	Muscle asymmetry
Lateral Bend	Muscle asymmetry
Rest Return	Return to rest level

Posture and Breathing Tests

Sitting Posture	Muscle symmetry
Deep Breathing	Muscle activity level
Standing Posture	Muscle symmetry
Deep Breathing	Muscle activity level

Muscle Length, Strength, Condition

	Length	Strength	Condition	EMG
Quadratus Lumborum				
Lumbar Paraspinals				
Abdominals				
Iliopsoas				
Pectineus				
Adductors				
Medial Rotators				
Lateral Rotators				
Adductors				
Piriformis				
Hamstrings				
Sartorius				
TFL				
Breathing Diaphragm				
Urogenital Diaphragm				
Pelvic Diaphragm				
Anal Sphincter				
Obturator Internus				

Figure 22 Muscle length, strength, condition chart

Palpation Assessment

Name:_____ Date:_____

                Grade   Comments

Resting:_____

Quck Contractions:_____

Hold Contractions:_____

Valsalva:_____

Other:_____

Observation:_____

Pelvic Muscle Strength Rating Scale:

	0	1	2	3
Pressure	None	Weak, feel pressure on side of fingers, but not all around	Moderate feel pressure all around	Strong, fingers compress/ override
Duration	None	<1 Second	1-3 Seonds	>3 Seconds
Displacement in plane	None	Slight incline, base of fingers moves up	Greater incline fingers move up along total length	Fingers move up and are drawn in

Figure 23 Pelvic Muscle Palpation Rating Scale & Assessment

Pelvic Muscle Force Field EMG Evaluation

A. Use of a Sensor

1. Use a personal vaginal, anal or surface sensor.

2. The individual empties bladder, then applies a small amount of lubricant to the top of the sensor before inserting the sensor in the vagina or rectum while standing with knees bent or semi-sitting or sidelying. Redress with the cord end outside the clothing. If surface sensors are used, clean the area with an alcohol pad.

3. When session is completed, remove the internal sensor, wash and rinse the sensor for 3 minutes under warm running water using mild soap, then air dry in sterile baggie. If surface sensors are used remove the surface sensors and dispose of the sensors and leads in a hazardous waste disposal.

B. Evaluation Components

1. Resting Level – sitting, supine, sidely or standing

2. Quick Contractions/Flicks
   This is a strong-fast contraction followed by an immediate relaxation. It primarily tests the urogenital diaphragm, fast acting fibers.

3. Ten Second Hold – 3 parts
   a. Isolated Hold of Pelvic Diaphragm – the average hold for someone who is leaking is 3-4 seconds without recruitment of accessory muscles.
   b. Roll Outs / Obturator Internus – against resistance roll legs out 2-4 inches and hold for a count of 10.
   c. Roll Ins / Adductors – against resistance bring legs together and hold for a count of 10.

4. Standing Plie – Bend the knees 2-3 inches for a count of 5 then straighten them for a count of 5 with feet pointed out.

C. Report:

1. Amplitude of contraction
2. Duration of contraction
3. Latency to peak of contraction
4. Latency to return to rest
5. Accessory muscles used: abdominals, gluteals, breath holding
6. Comparison of amplitude and duration of three types of 10 sec. holds
7. Resting level characteristics

EMG Assessment

Name:_____ Date: _____

POSITION: supine, sit, sidely, stand   ELECTRODE TYPE: surface, vaginal, anal

	Pelvic / Urogenital Diaphragm Muscles Comments		Other _____	
	Gross	Net	Gross	Net
1. Resting:				
2.Quick Contractions:				
3. Isolated Hold Contractions:				
4. Assisted Hold Obturators:				
5. Assisted Hold Adductors:				
6. Standing Rest:				
7. Standing Isolated:				
8. Standing Plie:				

*Net contractions = gross contraction amplitude minus resting level amplitude.
+Comments = observations of breath holding, associated muscle use, etc.

Thermal Assessment

Right:_____ Left:_____ Sensor Type:_____

Breathing Assessment

Sensor Type:_____

Description: _____

Problem List

1. _____
2. _____
3. _____
4. _____

Figure 24 Biofeedback Assessment Pelvic Muscle Force Field

Name_____ Date_____

Age_____ Sex_____ Therapist _____

ELECTRODE PLACEMENT

Site 1 _____ Site 2 _____

STRESS PROFILE

	EMG1	EMG2	Temp 1	Temp2
Baseline	_____	_____	_____	_____
Math	_____	_____	_____	_____
Recovery	_____	_____	_____	_____
Stress Story	_____	_____	_____	_____
Recovery	_____	_____	_____	_____
Pain Story	_____	_____	_____	_____
Recovery	_____	_____	_____	_____

DYNAMIC EVALUATION

	EMG1	EMG2
Baseline	_____	_____
Flexion	_____	_____
Rest	_____	_____
Ⓛ ROT	_____	_____
Rest	_____	_____
Ⓡ ROT	_____	_____
Rest	_____	_____
Ⓛ LAT Bend	_____	_____
Rest	_____	_____
Ⓡ LAT Bend	_____	_____

A.D.L.

_____   _____ _____
_____   _____ _____
_____   _____ _____
_____   _____ _____

Figure 25 Neuromuscular Assessment

POSTURAL EVALUATION

	L	R
sit		
breathe		
stand		
breathe		
supine/recline		
breathe		

PHYSIOLOGICAL QUIETING

	L	R
breathing		
support		
handwarming		
muscular - face		
head/neck		
back		
left arm		
right arm		
left leg		
right leg		
abdomen & chest		
final		

INTERPRETIVE COMMENTS

Figure 25 Neuromuscular assessment

Pelvic Muscle Rehab Treatment Plan

Name:_____ Age:_____ Initial Visit:_____

Referring MD: _____ Treatment Plan Completed: ☐Yes ☐No

Chief Complaint: _____
_____

Patient's Goals:

    1. _____
    2. _____
    3. _____

History:

_____
_____
_____
_____
_____

Assessment:

_____
_____
_____
_____
_____

Intervention:

_____
_____
_____
_____

Outcome Criteria:

_____
_____
_____

Discharge / Maintenance Evaluation:

_____
_____

Clinicians's Signature _____

Figure 26 Treatment Plan

Chapter 13

Additional Tests and Considerations

Physiological Tests

Self tests that indicate the status of underlying physiological processes indicate how well the automatic control centers of the body are functioning to allow pain free, fatigue free work and daily activities. These include blood glucose levels, blood pressure and heart rate, breathing pattern rate, and basal body temperature. Rather than working until the pain or fatigue prevents function, it is now often possible to test certain physiological processes and make adjustments so pain and fatigue do not become the prevalent aspect of each day. It is necessary to have testable signs that lead to appropriate intervention on a daily, sometimes even hourly basis.

Basic Self Tests	New Self Tests
■ Pain Level	■ Blood Glucose Level
■ Fatigue Level	■ Basal Body Temperature
■ Sleep Patterns	■ Blood Pressure
■ Work Duration	■ Heart Rate
■ Tender/Trigger Points	■ Breathing Pattern/Rate

Combining the Basic Self Tests and the New Self Tests provides an unprecedented compilation of data about the inner workings of each individual with CPP. Using this information it is possible to respond more specifically and appropriately with interventions to prevent symptoms. When these tests are done on a frequent basis the interventions can occur before the imbalance of physiological processes lead to limiting symptoms.

Baseline testing for 2-3 days can include all tests or only specific ones. Those tests that are indicative of imbalances for that individual are then placed in the Personal Profile Summary. (Figure 28) Each individual will have his/her own Key Indicator Tests. For Mary, her Key Indicator Tests included sleep patterns and basal body temperature. For Sue the list included blood glucose and blood pressure. Both individuals also monitored pain and fatigue levels.

Pick 2-3 days that you are able to concentrate on your own needs. Then follow the Baseline Testing Procedure for Chronic Pelvic Pain.

Baseline Testing Procedure for Chronic Pelvic Pain

First complete the General Criteria Questionnaire for Chronic Pelvic Pain. (Figure 16) Include Associated Symptoms and Patterns and Variations. (Figure 17) Then complete the Self Care Report (Figure 21) and Work/Rest Cycle (Figure 18) for 1-2 days. Summarize the results. Then proceed to the Key Indicator Tests below.

Key Indicator Tests of CPP Subcategories

The Key Indicators Tests provide information about the body's physiological status. Perform the Key Indicator Tests for one to two days. Record the results on the Daily Record Sheet. (Figure 27) Once this has been completed, interpret your results.

Blood Glucose

Equipment: use a blood glucose monitor. Follow the instructions on the unit. A blood glucose monitor can be purchased at a pharmacy.

Technique: Test your blood glucose level six times per day for 1-2 days and record the results on the daily nutrition and glucose level chart.

- on awakening each morning
- prior to each meal
- 1 hour after each meal
- 3 hours after each meal if another meal has not been eaten prior to going to bed

It is very important that you record everything you eat and drink on the daily nutrition and glucose level chart and place the items on the hour when they are eaten. This enables a comparison of types of food eaten with glucose levels. Also, record how you feel mentally and physically at the time of each test.

Basal Body Temperature

Equipment: Oral thermometer.

Technique: In the morning before getting out of bed take your oral or underarm temperature. Before lunch and dinner and at bedtime record your oral or underarm temperature.

Heart Rate and Blood Pressure

Equipment: A heart rate and blood pressure monitor. Follow the instructions on the unit. A blood pressure monitor can be purchased at a pharmacy.

Technique: Test your heart rate and blood pressure five times during the day. In the morning before you get out of bed, after breakfast, at lunch, at dinner, and before bedtime.

Breathing Pattern/Rate

Equipment: A watch with second hand, pen and paper.

Technique: Three times a day record your breathing pattern and rate for 1-2 minutes. For 15 seconds count the number of breaths and multiply by 4 to obtain the breaths per minute. Note where your breathing is occurring – in your abdomen, in your chest, in your neck and shoulders. Record all areas where you feel movement and breath on the daily breathing record sheet.

Daily Record Sheet

	Blood Pressure Rate	Blood Glucose Food Eaten	Basal Body Temp	Breathing Rate/ Location
Day 1				
Day 2				
Day 3				

Interpretation Record:

1. _____

2. _____

3. _____

Figure 27 Daily Record Sheet

INTERPRETING THE TESTS

Blood Glucose Level

The glucose level in the blood is the sugar level in the blood that is available to interact with insulin and then be used by all cells of the body for energy. Normal blood glucose level is considered to be 80-120mg/dl. Clinical observation indicates optimal function for individuals with hypoglycemic or reactive hypoglycemic tendencies is 95 to 120 mg/dl. Optimal function of the body and mind occur between these levels. To maintain this level throughout the day insulin from the pancreas must be given off into the blood stream at a variable rate depending on many factors including the level of exercise, stress and the amount and type of food eaten. If too much insulin is given off it breaks down excessive blood sugar and the blood glucose level drops below the normal levels. This can be termed hypoglycemia or reactive hypoglycemia. If too little insulin is given off there remains too high a level of sugar in the blood stream since the small amount of insulin can combine with only a small portion of glucose. This is termed high blood glucose levels and can be indicative of diabetes. The symptoms of low blood sugar or hypoglycemia often include irritability, irrationality, physical fatigue, and muscle weakness. Additionally, as the reaction progresses sweating, increase in heart rate, dizziness and lightheadedness, mental confusion, emotional outbursts, and extreme anxiety occur. Anger and resistance to others' suggestions is common. These symptoms are the result of low sugar (food) available to the brain, voluntary and autonomic nervous systems, and muscles.

Record the blood glucose levels in the daily record sheet using a glucometer and the blood from your knee or finger. Consult with your health care professional about the technique for using a glucometer.

Record the food you eat and the time you eat so a comparison can be made between the blood glucose reading and the type and amount of food you have taken in. During the days of record keeping engage in your normal physical exercise that is part of your daily routine. Be sure to indicate when and how much you exercise since this can affect blood glucose levels.

Interpret Your Results

Looking at the data, ask yourself, "Is my blood glucose stable throughout the day or is there a large variation?" "Does my blood glucose level tend to be in the 80s or below, 80s and 90s, or 95 and above?" "Does my blood glucose level ever go over 140?" "What do I feel like and what are the symptoms I am experiencing when my blood glucose test results are in the 80s or below? In the 90s, over 95?"

Basal Body Temperature

Basal body temperature is the heat created by the body's metabolism (fire). Normal basal body temperature is 98.6° F. If the body's metabolism is very low the body temperature will be decreased. If metabolism is high the body temperature will be increased. Heat is created within each cell of the body and is the result of the conversion of nutrients and chemicals into cellular energy. Even a small change in temperature affects cellular function significantly. Blood releases oxygen to the cells more readily at warmer temperatures and more slowly at cooler temperatures. Extreme temperature changes are life threatening. A decrease in body temperature to 97.6° F is significant enough to change physical and mental processes. The feeling of being cold, cold hands and feet, alternately feeling hot and cold, or sweating and shivering are common symptoms. Pain and mental confusion occur with longer term temperature decrease. More familiar are the symptoms associated with increased body temperature of which sweating and feeling hot are the most common symptoms. Fatigue and lethargy occur with fever as well.

Interpret Your Results

Record your basal body temperatures at predetermined times. Ask these questions:

"Is my temperature lower or higher than the normal 98.6° F? If it is different is it consistently lower or higher or only at certain times of the day? How do I feel – cold, hot, energized, fatigued, painful, pain free?" Record a summary in the Interpretation Record.

Blood Pressure/ Heart Rate

Blood pressure is the force of the blood traveling out of the heart and down the arteries of the body. Normal blood pressure for adults less than 60 years old is 120/80mm/hg. Consistent readings above 150/90mm/hg are considered high blood pressure. Consistent readings below 100/70mm/hg is considered low blood pressure. 120mm/hg is the pressure of the ventricle pushing the blood into the ascending aorta, 80mm/hg is the pressure in the blood vessel in between beats. Heart rate at rest averages 60-70 beats per minute (bpm) on the average. Resting heart rate above 90 beats per minute is considered excessive. Blood pressure and heart rate are controlled to a large extent by the autonomic nervous system. Record your blood pressure and heart rate in the daily record sheet.

Interpret Your Results

Answer the questions, " Is my heart rate above 90 bpm at rest? Is my blood pressure normal, high or low? Does my blood pressure and/or heart rate change with different positions? Does my blood pressure or heart rate vary greatly or remain stable?" Record your comments in the Interpretation Report including any symptoms you or those around you perceive as occurring when you take your blood pressure and heart rate.

Breathing Pattern/Rate

An individual's breathing is automatic and the pattern and rate are generally similar for everyone. At rest 10-12 breaths per minute is within normal limits. Breathing is designed to provide oxygen for use by the body cells in burning fuels for energy and function. It is designed to excrete waste products like carbon dioxide. Oxygen and carbon dioxide are essential for function but are toxic when present in excess. The acidity of the body is largely determined by the level of carbon dioxide in the blood stream. Virtually all metabolic processes depend on adequate acid-base balance. Increased carbon dioxide is correlated with nervous system hyperexcitability – muscles are hyperirritable, pupils dilate, extremities are cold, and there is increased sweating. During hyperventilation (shallow breathing with loss of carbon dioxide) blood flow to the brain, hands, feet, and intestines decreases. This can affect thinking and memory, digestion and absorption of food as well as coordination and ambulation. Hyperventilation has been linked to a sudden dramatic decrease in blood pressure which may result in syncope or fainting. Breathing also affects heart rate and cellular metabolism. Breathing is automatic, you do not have to think about each breath. If you had to think about each breath it would be hard to get anything else done during the day. During exercise your breathing rate increases and during meditation or sleep it decreases. Diaphragmatic breathing is the most efficient form of breathing. During diaphragmatic breathing, as you inhale your diaphragm descends and the abdomen will rise or move outward. As you exhale the diaphragm will return to the dome shape and the abdomen will move inward. The diaphragm is descending into the abdominal cavity with inhalation and ascending or rising towards the breastbone with exhale. During diaphragmatic breathing the upper chest and shoulders are quiet and the abdominal muscles are relatively relaxed. The jaw is released, the teeth separated, and the tongue is relaxed at the bottom of the mouth, the tip of the tongue resting lightly behind the top front teeth. Hyperventilation is characterized by rapid chest breathing. Irregular breathing cycles, sighing, and interrupted breathing (apnea) can also occur.

Interpret Your Results

Record the interpretation of your typical breathing noticing where the breathing occurs – in the neck, shoulders, chest, abdomen or diaphragm. If you noticed movement in your upper chest and/or shoulders during breathing the accessory muscles of neck and chest are being used for each breath. Then record the pattern of your breathing. Normal breathing pattern is equal inhale and exhale with slight rest between each. Ask yourself, "Do I inhale and exhale equally or is my inhale longer or shorter than my exhale?" "Do I yawn a lot? Do I feel out of breath at rest or doing quiet activities?" Yawning and shortness of breath may indicate an abnormal breathing pattern.

Is your breathing rate average, slower or faster than the average? Do you breathe using the breathing diaphragm or using the neck, chest and shoulder muscles? What is your breathing pattern – the inhale to exhale ratio? Record your interpretation of breathing pattern, rate, and location on the Interpretation Record.

Personal Profile Summary

My Major Characteristics & Associated Symptoms

1. _____
   _____

2. _____
   _____

3. _____
   _____

4. _____
   _____

5. _____
   _____

My Key Indicators:

1. _____
   _____

2. _____
   _____

3. _____
   _____

My Subcategories:

1. _____
   _____

2. _____
   _____

Figure 28 Personal Profile

Now it is possible to identify which tests indicated changes in your body function that relate to physical and mental symptoms labeled Chronic Pelvic Pain symptoms. List the Key Indicator Tests that indicate deviation from normal levels. Identify the physiological subcategory(ies) that are closest to your characteristics using the Key Indicators and the Physiological Subcategory Symptoms.

Physiological Subcategories
Neurally Mediated Hypotension Tendencies

Symptoms

Individuals with Neurally Mediated Hypotension Tendencies (NMH), also called vasomotor syncope, describe low blood pressure and high resting heart rate. Heart rate is often 90-100 beats per minute at rest when 60-70 is considered normal. Blood pressure is often 95/65 mm Hg when 110/70 is considered normal. These individuals in addition to CPP describe feeling weak in the knees, dizzy and light headed, especially when getting up from lying or sitting. They describe mental and physical fatigue. Additionally they describe chest pain that so closely imitates heart problems a physician may do a complete cardiac workup, yet find nothing. They describe problems with swallowing and indigestion. They describe shortness of breath with minimal exertion. They describe abdominal pain that closely imitates pain from gall stones, interstitial cystitis, endometriosis, or cancer.

Neurally Mediated Hypotension Symptoms
❑ Low Blood Pressure   ❑ Mental Fatigue
❑ High Resting Heart Rate   ❑ Chest Pain
❑ Dizzy / Light Headed   ❑ Difficulty Swallowing
❑ Weak

Case Studies

Linda had six abdominal surgeries in three years to find what was causing the extreme pain and dysfunction. She had her gall bladder, loops of her intestine, her uterus, ovaries, and scar tissue removed. Nothing helped and she was worse after the surgeries at the end of three years. Clearly something else was producing the abdominal pain.

Melissa described her legs melting from under her while she was shopping. She felt her heart racing at times even when she was resting. She tired easily and quickly during her attempts at exercise or during recreational activities. She experienced such extreme discomfort and bloating in her abdomen that she could not wear clothing that touched her stomach. She had bouts of constipation and diarrhea. She burped unpleasant gas and experienced indigestion and stomach pain to a point that she was afraid to eat. Changing her diet did not help. Her abdominal pain increased before her menstrual cycle to the point she would often be in bed for several days with pain, weakness, nausea and vomiting. Her menstrual cycle was regular within 7-10 days. During her menstrual cycle the uterine cramping was intense. She described frequent feelings of urgency to toilet, getting up 1-2 times nightly and toileting every 1-2 hours. Yet, at other times Melissa felt great, energetic, athletic, and pain free.

Etiology/Cause

Neurally mediated hypotension is often overlooked as a possible cause for the symptoms of abnormal heart rate and blood pressure, chest and abdominal pain. The ANS-HPA-RHA messaging systems are not working together effectively to normalize heart rate, blood pressure, muscle and organ function in NMH. There is nothing wrong structurally with any of the organ systems. Rather it is the messaging systems that tell them what to do and how to do it that are dysfunctional. These dysfunctional messaging systems may also affect the blood flow to the organs which can lead to further symptoms at the organ level.

Melissa and others like her give us clues about how to help the symptoms. She told us, "When I feel terrible, if I go to McDonald's and have french fries I feel a lot better even though I know they are not good for me. My energy improves, my weak knees disappear, and my diarrhea improves."

Before we knew much about the heart and gut regulation centers and their potential affects on the rest of the body, Melissa's comments were baffling. To understand why McDonald's french fries helped Melissa and others with CPP it is necessary to understand some facts about the heart and gut control centers.

Gut Absorption and Heart Function

The body's serotonin, 95% of which is produced by the enteric nervous system of the gut, affects all cells of the body with receptor sites for serotonin. When the gut produces an abundance of serotonin it flows not only in the gut influencing the function there, but also to the brain, to the heart, to the blood vessels, to the uterus, and to the bladder. In the gut serotonin facilitates peristalsis, in the heart it increases the heart rate, in the blood vessels it stimulates constriction, in the uterus and bladder it induces contraction, and in the brain it facilitates sleep and decreases pain perception. Thus, the gut's enteric nervous system is an essential component in treating and controlling CPP symptoms of high resting heart rate, low blood pressure and abdominal pain.

The gut's function is to digest food, absorb the digested nutrients into the blood stream and defend against poisons. The enteric nervous system controls the efficiency and effectiveness of these functions. It determines to a large extent what nutrients and how much of each nutrient is absorbed and how much is excreted in the feces/bowel movements. If salts from food are excreted in excess rather than being absorbed into the bloodstream, every cell of the body is affected in their ability to function optimally. Salts affect the dilation or constriction of blood vessels and the energy produced in muscle cells, just to mention two. A deficiency in sodium chloride salts results in blood vessel dilation, which results in the muscle we call the heart beating faster but less effectively, and in the skeletal muscles of the trunk, arms and legs contracting less effectively and relaxing incompletely. The human body can have a functionally low sodium chloride level that may or may not be detectable by the usual medical testing but the function of every cell of the body is affected by the lack of available salt. Increasing sodium chloride levels in the bloodstream so they are available to body cells will improve heart, blood vessel, and skeletal muscle function just to name a few.

Increasing sodium chloride in the diet of CPP individuals experiencing symptoms of high resting heart rate, low blood pressure, and abdominal pain may significantly improve the symptoms. When there is adequate sodium chloride, the blood vessels constrict/close more effectively which increases the pressure of the blood as it travels through them. Normal blood pressure results. The heart, in response to increased sodium chloride levels, slows the number of beats per minute and the pumping function becomes more effective and efficient. The skeletal muscles of the trunk, arms and legs are able to contract and relax quickly and completely in repetitive fashion when they have adequate sodium chloride. The muscle cells are thus able to receive the nutrients they need from the blood and lymph and can rid themselves of waste products effectively. Weakness, fatigue, pain, and stiffness decrease in the individual with CPP when there is adequate sodium chloride available to the cells.

Serotonin and Gut Pain

The enteric nervous system in CPP seems to oscillate between the extremes of activity or fatigue instead of holding to a middle ground of stimulating activity and rest. There is no balanced work-rest cycle. One example is the serotonin release by the enteric nervous system. Serotonin is released when there is pressure on the bowel lining cells. The serotonin excites peristalsis and thus elimination. If in the CPP gut the release of serotonin is excessive the peristalsis is initially increased which could cause diarrhea, dehydration and discomfort. As the serotonin continues to flow it "drowns" the magnet receptor sites in the gut and as with any drowning victim the sites cease to function so the gut shuts down. Excessive serotonin results in paralysis of the gut until the excess serotonin is broken down or otherwise incapacitated. Constipation and even impaction with inflammation results when the gut shuts down. Pain is present. Constipation and impaction of the gut is accompanied by abdominal pain, inability to stand up straight and a shuffling gait with quick fatigue. In severe cases, the individual cannot get up from a chair without help.

Improving the enteric nervous system function in the gut of CPP individuals experiencing symptoms of high resting heart rate, low blood pressure, and abdominal pain may significantly improve the symptoms.

When there is dysfunction or imbalance of the enteric system every other organ system in the body is potentially dysfunctional as well. The enteric nervous system communicates with the heart via the vagus nerve complex, it communicates with the pancreas which produces insulin via enteric peripheral nerves and information chemicals, it communicates with uterus and bladder much the same way. If the enteric nervous system is in a high activation mode the gut will transfer food from mouth to anus faster than usual. Additionally the uterus and the bladder can be more irritable, and the heart can beat faster. As a result, the muscles of the body receive oxygen and food products at a different rate and amount. The muscle cell metabolism is changed. Waste product removal is altered. The entire body is affected when the enteric nervous system of the gut is dysfunctional.

Testing

The diagnosis of NMH tendencies is most often based on a medical history, symptom diary and heart rate/blood pressure tests. If the symptoms are appropriate, the heart rate relatively elevated and/or the blood pressure low, NMH is considered as a subcategory type in CPP. There is a medical test to diagnose autonomic neurally mediated hypotension as this category is termed by some physicians. It is the tilt table test usually performed by a cardiologist. The individual is placed on a tilt table, a table that has a foot rest and can be tilted from horizontal to vertical position in varying degrees. The table is tilted 70 degrees from horizontal for 45 minutes. The blood pools in the feet unless the heart works adequately and the veins in the legs and abdomen have adequate tone to push the blood back up to the heart and brain. When the autonomic nervous system is not responsive to the stress of the tilt the blood pressure drops and the heart rate does not increase adequately to keep the blood from pooling in the feet. The individual experiences widespread pain, fainting, nausea and even vomiting. Some individuals pass out. The sequelae may last several days after the test. Since the test is so aversive, it is not usually done until the individual tries a self care treatment approach and still has significant symptoms.

To determine if a food intolerance is part of the problem it is recommended that the individual eliminate that food product from the diet for 7-10 days and document any relief in symptoms. If the relief is significant then a change in diet is recommended.

Hypoglycemic Tendencies

Symptoms

In addition to CPP, these individuals describe feeling shaky, dizzy, irritable, irrational and weak. Other symptoms include headache, depression, anxiety, sweets cravings, confusion, night sweats, and insomnia. These individuals can become aggressive and easily lose their tempers during a hypoglycemic episode. Stress increases the levels of stress hormones. Stress hormones increase metabolism, activate insulin release, and increase glucose utilization.

Even though the standard definition of hypoglycemia is a blood sugar level below 50 mg/dl, in recent years there have been several studies that suggest individuals have different set points for blood sugar. When there is a drop below the individual's specific set point the brain and body exhibit "I'm in trouble" signs. The set point in the research studies varied from the 50s to the 80s. That means that an CPP individual could have a high set point in the 70s or 80s and exhibit symptoms of muscle stiffness, cramping and weakness, fatigue, irritability, insomnia, and mental confusion due to "hypoglycemic tendencies." The patient's history and symptoms will provide the best indication of this subtype of CPP although blood sugar levels can be of help if there is an acceptance that symptoms and set points are the criteria, not a blood glucose reading of 50.

Hypoglycemia Symptoms

- ☐ Hunger Shakes/Tremors
- ☐ Fainting
- ☐ Heart Palpitations
- ☐ Irregular Heart Beats
- ☐ Panic Attacks
- ☐ Anxiety
- ☐ Sweats

- ☐ Fatigue
- ☐ Sleep Disturbance
- ☐ Blurred Vision
- ☐ Gut Pain, Gas
- ☐ Headaches
- ☐ Memory/Concentration Problems

Case Study

Linda's husband describes her as the sweetest, most giving person he has ever met, yet he comments that she has a tendency to snap and blow up at any little thing. He notes that she frequently complains of pain in her shoulders, neck and head as well as her CPP. She sometimes wakes him up at night in a sweat. These symptoms began after the birth of their first child so they assumed it was just a readjustment from pregnancy. Now two years later they are both concerned that the symptoms haven't gone away. Her physician diagnosed CPP and the medications have helped some but she still experiences fatigue, pain, and mood changes that have a rapid onset, i.e. one minute she's feeling good and the next she feels lousy.

Etiology/Cause

Hypoglycemia is a condition of low blood glucose (sugar) levels with resulting symptoms. Any or all of the symptoms may occur as quickly as 30-60 minutes after a meal or as long as 2-3 hours after eating. For some reason there is an imbalance between insulin and glucose in the blood stream which leads to the low blood sugar.

The two subtypes of hypoglycemia are:

- General Hypoglycemia
- Reactive Hypoglycemia

The two subtypes are differentiated by 1) the time frame between eating and the onset of low blood sugar and 2) the type of food that sets off the symptoms. In General Hypoglycemia the onset of hypoglycemic symptoms is usually 2-3 hours after a meal. In Reactive Hypoglycemia the onset of symptoms is more immediate, usually 30-60 minutes after eating. In the case of General Hypoglycemia the foods that set off the symptoms include simple sugars and carbohydrates but not complex carbohydrates. In the case of Reactive Hypoglycemia complex carbohydrates as well as simple sugars and carbohydrates can set off the symptoms.

- General Hypoglycemia   2-3 hrs. simple sugars/carbos
- Reactive Hypoglycemia   1/2-1 hr. complex carbos
                                                      simple sugars/carbos

Both the time between eating and symptoms and the type of food eaten relate to the release of insulin and glucose (sugar) into the blood stream. This model for hypoglycemia takes into consideration the timing of insulin release from the pancreas and the timing of glucose release from the small intestine. The model also takes into consideration the amount of insulin or glucose released within a set amount of time, it could be a large amount (bolus) released in a short time period or smaller amounts (timed release capsules) over a 3-4 hour segment.

- General Hypoglycemia   Bolus insulin and glucose released in 1-2 hours symptoms experienced
- Reactive Hypoglycemia   Premature bolus of insulin released Timed released glucose 1/2-1 hour symptoms experienced

Both hypoglycemia subtypes experience excessive movement of insulin and glucose into the blood stream (the sugar high) depleting the glucose available in a short amount of time in response to simple sugars/carbohydrates. The result is low blood sugar (the crash). Reactive hypoglycemia differs in that it is also sensitive to complex carbohydrates which stimulate excessive and premature release of insulin. Both hypoglycemia subtypes are stimulated by stress, excessive exercise, caffeine or alcohol.

The cause of General Hypoglycemia is based on a dysfunctional glucose absorption model. Glucose is absorbed abnormally from the small intestine into the blood stream. The small intestine is the primary area of the gastrointestinal tract where nutrients are absorbed. If sugars are absorbed more slowly than insulin is released, low blood sugar results – hypoglycemia. The blood sugar and insulin are not balanced in the blood stream. The enteric nervous system controls sugar absorption from the gut to the blood stream and release of insulin from the pancreas. When the enteric brake is "on" the gut slows or even stops the absorption of nutrients into the blood stream. When the enteric brake is "off" the gut speeds up the absorption of nutrients into the blood stream. The enteric brake is stimulated to be "off" when sugars and simple carbohydrates enter the stomach. In General Hypoglycemia the enteric brake is "off" so the gut sends sugars to the blood stream and the pancreas sends insulin into the blood stream more rapidly than normal. Within a 2-3 hour period the available glucose is utilized and blood sugar levels drop. The CPP individual with general hypoglycemic tendencies exhibits symptoms that interfere with their daily life when blood sugar levels drop into the 70/80 range or below.

The cause of Reactive Hypoglycemia is based on an abnormal insulin release model. Insulin is released prematurely and excessively by the pancreas. In Reactive Hypoglycemia, when simple or complex carbohydrates are chewed and swallowed, the enteric nervous system sends messages to the pancreas telling it to immediately release insulin into the bloodstream at a rapid rate and in substantial amounts. Meanwhile, the carbohydrate now in the gut is taking hours to be digested and then absorbed into the bloodstream. The insulin looks for the great quantity of sugar (glucose) that the enteric nervous system said would be waiting for it in the bloodstream and finds relatively little. It combines with any glucose available but finds little. This imbalance of insulin versus glucose in the bloodstream leads to a rapid depletion of blood glucose resulting in the symptoms of shakiness, confusion, pain, fatigue and agitation within 30-60 minutes of eating. The organ systems i.e., the brain, muscles, blood vessels are not getting the consistent level of glucose combined with insulin they need to function normally.

Testing

The first assessment is a review of symptoms by the individual and a close family member or friend (See Symptoms, page 124). The involvement of a family member or friend is important because the individual may not be aware of all the external appearances of symptoms if the hypoglycemia is moderate to severe. Individuals with long term hypoglycemia may assume the symptoms are normal feelings.

When the symptom review is completed the next step is to monitor blood glucose levels periodically throughout the day for 1-2 days. It is important to also keep track of the food eaten at each meal and snack and any symptoms you are experiencing at the time of the blood glucose reading. Blood glucose readings every one to two hours can differentiate between General and Reactive Hypoglycemic tendencies. Blood glucose readings should be done:

- on awakening each morning
- prior to each meal
- 1 hour after each meal
- 3 hours after each meal if another meal has not been eaten
- prior to going to bed

Optimal blood glucose range is 90-120. Below 90 individuals can begin to experience symptoms and by the time an individual reaches 80 they describe feeling significant symptoms. In the 60-70 range work and self care function is severely affected.

To differentiate between subtypes monitor the blood glucose readings after a high carbohydrate meal and then after a high protein/fat meal. Assess how quickly the symptoms occur after eating. Fatigue, pain and personality changes within 30 minutes to one hour after eating a high carbohydrate meal is more likely Reactive Hypoglycemia. Fatigue, pain and personality changes 2-3 hours after a meal relatively high in simple sugars/carbohydrates is more likely General Hypoglycemia.

It is important to test immediately on awakening and as you go to bed each night. Hypoglycemia can occur at night as well as during the day. If blood sugar is low as you go to bed at night and/or low when you first wake up in the morning the implication is that you are experiencing hypoglycemic tendencies during the night. Sleep disturbance and night sweats are common with night time hypoglycemia.

A glucose tolerance test (GTT) performed in a medical center can indicate hypoglycemia. The individual is required to fast for 12 hours and then glucose is given in measured doses. The test is usually done over 5 hours testing the level of glucose in the blood each hour. If glucose levels are low or erratic the diagnosis is hypoglycemia. Some individuals will have normal test results but still experience symptoms.

Case Study

Mary, a 45 year old teacher, describes having CPP for the past 4 years since a hysterectomy. On awakening in the morning she is stiff and sore so she immediately takes a hot shower and does some stretching to get ready for the day. Her usual breakfast before going to work is a bowl of oatmeal with raisins and brown sugar, 2 slices of toast with butter and jam, a large glass of orange juice and 2 cups of coffee. Her husband states she comes to the breakfast table in a good mood but after breakfast she usually has something nasty to say and sometimes forgets her keys and lunch as she leaves. Mary says that after breakfast she feels more tired physically and mentally than before breakfast. She doesn't understand how that could be.

In Mary's case the high carbohydrate breakfast stimulates an immediate and large release of insulin into the blood stream. The carbohydrates are still primarily in the stomach while the insulin pours into the blood stream and combines with any glucose it can find. The result is the blood glucose levels drop significantly and quickly. Within 30 minutes Mary was feeling "lousy" because her blood sugar was too low and she would go back to bed if she could.

Individuals like Mary feel better, have more energy and less pain, and an improved personality when they eat eggs or meat for breakfast. Mary remembers times during the work day when she felt shaky and tired. If she stopped by McDonald's and got a Big Mac she felt better quickly. Was this just a break from work or did Big Macs have a miraculous quality? The high protein in the Big Mac doesn't trigger the large insulin release.

Hypothyroid Tendencies

Symptoms

Symptoms of hypothyroid tendencies include feeling cold, cold hands and feet, feeling core cold at times, weight gain, dry skin, heavy menstruation, PMS, and constipation. Additional complaints include fatigue, sleep disturbance, and stiff achiness rather than sharp pains. These descriptors may be from hypothyroid tendencies, a sluggish thyroid gland that is not producing adequate thyroid hormone or dysfunction of thyroid hormone at the cellular level. Thyroid hormone produced by the thyroid gland is an essential information molecule for many body functions. Another essential thyroid hormone is produced primarily at the cellular tissue level using a hormone originating in the thyroid gland.

Hypothyroid Symptoms

☐ Muscle Weakness
☐ Excess Sleepiness
☐ Weight Gain
☐ Constipation
☐ Digestive Problems
☐ Cold Intolerance
☐ Body Temperature
    Below 97.6° F

☐ Menstrual Irregularities
☐ Hoarse, Deep Voice
☐ Memory/Concentration
    Problems
☐ Depression
☐ Hair Loss
☐ Dry Skin

Case Study

Margaret, a 35-year-old mother of three, complained to her health care professional about severe fatigue, overall stiffness and aching, headaches, PMS, weight gain, and a core feeling of cold as well as CPP. She began to crave chocolate bars and coke. Her thyroid function tests were normal but her basal body temperature was decreased. Her thyroid hormone T4 to T3 conversion was dysfunctional at the cellular level.

Etiology/Cause

Many times an individual with CPP complains of these "hypothyroid tendency" symptoms but the thyroid function test is normal. There is another form of thyroid chemical dysfunction that cannot be measured by blood tests. The symptoms have been documented in the medical literature since the 1970s. For our purposes this dysfunction will be termed cell level hypothyroidism.

Cell Level Problem

Cell level hypothyroidism is abnormal cellular T4 to T3 conversion. In other words the thyroid hormone T4 flows from the thyroid gland into the blood stream and then to magnet sites on body cells, for example to magnet sites on muscle cells. There T4 must be converted to T3 to be of use to the muscle cell in energy production. If that conversion does not take place, or is sluggish or incomplete, cell level hypothyroidism may result. Inadequate T3 at the cellular level can lead to stiffness, achiness, a decrease in basal body temperature, constipation and dry skin. T3 is essential for cell metabolism – lighting and maintaining the fire that produces energy in the cell. When the fire is hard to light, of low intensity, or erratic, outward symptoms appear.

An individual may have dysfunction at the thyroid level and at the cellular level simultaneously. In this case treating the thyroid level deficiency will alleviate some symptoms but the cellular level treatment will be necessary for more complete relief of symptoms.

Basic Physiology

To review thyroid function and its hormonal importance to body function we begin with the brain (Figure 29). The hypothalamus stimulates the pituitary gland in the brain which stimulates the thyroid gland in the neck region to produce T4 (Thyroxine). T4 is the foundation chemical needed to make the active thyroid chemical messenger T3 (Triiodothyronine). Approximately 80% of T3 formation occurs in the body cells not in the thyroid gland. T4 travels to the body cells via the blood stream so it can be measured in a blood test. T3 is produced in the tissue cells and remains there for the most part so a blood test does not indicate its level of production or effectiveness. T3 instructs body cells how fast or slow to operate and how hot the burners should be set to fire up the cellular activity. As such T3 is a major determinant of body temperature. A cell's burner is set high or low by T3. The test for T3 is Basal Body Temperature, the internal temperature of the body.

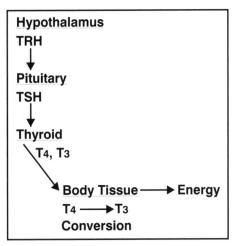

Figure 29 Thyroid Hormones

Metabolism and Temperature

Body temperature affects the overall metabolism of the body because the body's metabolism is the sum total of all the chemical reactions occurring in each cell. These chemical reactions are dependent on enzymes which are the "sparks of life." There are digestive enzymes and metabolic enzymes. Think of chemical reactions in cells as the fire that provides energy for the cell motor to run. Metabolic enzymes are the catalyst or stimulus that ignite the fire and helps determine the intensity of the fire. When temperature is decreased the enzymes are cold and stiff so the motor doesn't start easily, it sputters and runs only on one or two cylinders, quitting easily. When the temperature is increased, as when an individual has an illness with a high fever, the enzymes are too hot so the motor function is abnormal, at times to the point of destruction. When temperature is decreased the cells go into a form of hibernation, when the temperature is increased greatly the cells burn up from an explosion of energy. The basal body temperature is designed to be 98.6°F, just the right temperature for the enzymes to act effectively and efficiently in the metabolic burn. In this state the cell motor can be active at a balanced steady state for long periods of time without fatigue, pain, or depletion of essential elements. The body is able to provide the nutrients the cell needs for its motor function and remove the waste products at a rate that is conducive to long term function. The individual feels warm, feels energetic, and feels pain free and alert. The skin is in a healthy state, the nervous system is healthy and the reproductive system is able to function in a healthy state.

We know that changes in body temperature change body functions. The body goes into a conservation mode when body temperature decreases. It ceases to provide energy production except where it is needed for vital organs. The skin becomes dry, hair becomes brittle and falls out, and the reproductive system becomes dysfunctional. In the extreme, cells are destroyed and eventually organs die. Cell level hypothyroid tendency is experienced as a complex of symptoms brought on in part by alteration in body temperature.

Reproductive Hormones and Metabolism

The reproductive system affects thyroid function. Estrogen and progesterone facilitate thyroid function including the conversion of T4 to T3 at the cellular level. If estrogen/progesterone levels are decreased or the estrogen to progesterone ratio is abnormal there can be resultant changes in T4 to T3 conversion that will change the Basal Body Temperature and also result in cell level hypothyroid tendency symptoms.

ANS and Metabolism

The ANS significantly affects thyroid function. The enteric division determines the effective breakdown of protein, fat and carbohydrate nutrients to amino acids, fatty acids and sugars that the thyroid system can use in its synthesis and conversion of thyroid hormones. The sympathetic and parasympathetic divisions affect head brain function of the pituitary and hypothalamus glands that send messages to the thyroid. Both sympathetic and parasympathetic divisions send messages directly to the thyroid gland itself.

The Amino Acid Necklaces

The thyroid hormones are amino acid necklaces. The protein we eat is broken down in the intestines into 20-30 amino acids some of which combine to form the thyroid hormones T4 and T3. Protein contains approximately 16 percent nitrogen while the other basic nutrients, sugars and fatty acids, contain no nitrogen. Amino acid necklaces form the chemical messengers that transfer messages between nerve cells as well as facilitate the metabolism, the motor in each body cell. Lysine is an essential amino acid that aids in production of enzymes within the cell body as one of its functions. Tyrosine is an essential amino acid that is a precursor to norepinephrine the parasympathetic nervous system messenger. It is a vital ingredient in the function of the thyroid gland, the adrenal glands and the pituitary gland. Tyrosine attaches to iodine to form active thyroid hormones including T3. Symptoms of low tyrosine can include low body temperature, weight gain, low blood pressure, restless leg syndrome, depression and anxiety.

Blood Sugar and Metabolism

Blood sugar levels also affect cell level hypothyroid tendencies and body temperature. Low blood sugar or hypoglycemia, decreases body temperature and decreases metabolism. A diabetic with low blood sugar experiences cold sweats and uncontrolled shivering. High blood sugar levels increase the body's temperature and increases metabolism which can lead to hot sweats. Symptoms of hypoglycemia are very similar to cellular hypothyroidism.

HPA Axis and Metabolism

Cortisol levels also affect body temperature. Cortisol is produced by the adrenal glands and is part of the "stress" hormone package. High cortisol levels decrease body temperature and inhibit the conversion of T4 to T3 leading to cellular hypothyroidism. Use of cortisone can also lead to the same symptoms.

Test

The first assessment is a review of symptoms by the individual and a close family member or friend. (See Symptoms, page 129) A blood test can determine the level of thyroid hormone produced by the thyroid gland in an individual. The blood test does not indicate the level of T3 available at the cellular level because the great majority of T3 is converted from T4 at the site of metabolic activity.

To test for cell level hypothyroid tendencies use an oral thermometer and place it under your arm or in your mouth for 15 minutes while you remain quiet. If the temperature is 97.6° F or below, it can indicate an underactive T4 to T3 conversion level. Barnes recommended taking the temperature on awakening before getting up from bed. Wilson recommends taking it 3 times a day approximately 3 hours apart during the times of the day when symptoms usually occur. So if fatigue, pain, and coldness occur in the afternoon more than in the morning the tests would be predominately done from noon on.

Body temperature changes cyclically through the day in both sexes and through the month in females. It is usually lowest in the morning, highest in the afternoon and then decreases as the evening progresses. Additionally, for women, estrogen and progesterone, the information molecules from the ovaries cause variations in body temperature as they cycle during the month. Body temperature rises at ovulation (day 14) and just prior to the menstrual period. Temperature changes on the day of ovulation and three days before the menstrual period starts are not as accurate as during the rest of the month in diagnosing cell level hypothyroidism.

Reproductive Hormone Imbalance Tendency

Symptoms

One category of symptoms described by individuals with CPP can be termed Reproductive Hormonal Imbalance Tendencies. These individuals describe monthly and/or yearly cycles of muscle pain, fatigue, sleep disturbance, menstrual irregularities, bowel and bladder irritability and depression.

Mary, as we described in the introduction, experienced incapacitating symptoms of body pain, fatigue, abdominal bloating, and gut dysfunction by Thanksgiving every year. She would miss work and school and would be in bed much of the time due to weakness and fatigue. Mentally she was depressed and when she tried to work she found she made many mistakes. She would try medications and food elimination without help. Using phytoestrogen and progesterone creams she was able to return to work and attend school. She did not become ill or need to limit her activities any more than other times of the year. She states she has confidence that her life is under more control and balance.

Joann described extreme symptoms the week before her menstrual cycle. She experienced fatigue, muscle pain, shakiness, and sleep disturbances. The abdominal pain at the beginning of menstruation incapacitated her for 1-3 days. She began using flax seed in her smoothie each morning and used phytoestrogen during the first 14 days and progesterone during the end of the month. Her menstrual cycle became more regular and the pain and fatigue along with the sleep disturbance improved to the point she was not missing work or school. She described her energy level and optimism improving to the point she would plan trips away from home during the week before her menstrual cycle was to begin.

Cause/Etiology

Estrogen and progesterone hormones (chemical messengers) produced primarily in the ovaries, affect all organ systems including the head brain, the gut brain, and the smooth and striated muscles. Estrogen facilitates the build up of edometrium in the uterus. It tends to increase blood pressure. Additionally estrogen facilitates sleep, a sense of well being, increased energy, increased endorphins (the natural body endorphins), and increased serotonin. It facilitates absorption of calcium through the intestine and increased blood flow to the brain and muscles. It facilitates thyroid hormone conversion of T4-T3. Progesterone facilitates slowing of the digestive system and tranquilizing mood, it increases appetite, sex drive, increases water retention in the body, facilitates breast engorgement and decreases blood pressure.

Estrogen and progesterone levels vary on a monthly (28 day) cycle in females. Estrogen rises more than progesterone during the first 14 days of the cycle. At ovulation estrogen and progesterone decline for several days. After ovulation, progesterone rises more than estrogen for the last 14 days. Then both decline with the initiation of the menses (period).

Reproductive hormones influence the circuitry in the central nervous system and the way the brain processes information. Hormonal changes that occur during the menstrual cycle can have profound effects on the way information is integrated in the central and peripheral nervous system. In one study testing ischemic pain (pain from lack of blood circulation), women expressed increased pain levels during the last 14 days of the menstrual cycle compared to the first 14 days. The last 14 days of the menstrual cycle are associated with higher levels of estrogen, progesterone and lutenizing hormones (female hormones). The masculinizing hormones known as the androgynous hormones are minimized in their effect during this time. Adrongenous hormones minimize pain perception compared to female hormones which accentuate pain perception. Maixner also found suppression of opiod induced systems during the same period of time (the last 14 days of the menstrual cycle may be related to opiod levels).

Estrogen/progesterone levels can affect muscle strength. Some females lose as much as 9-10% of muscle strength during the week before the period starts.

Estrogen and progesterone also vary on a yearly cycle. Estrogen and progesterone fall in the winter and rise in the summer. With transition times in the fall and spring. Estrogen and progesterone are at their highest level April through July and at their lowest from October through January. This may help to explain reports of increased CPP during winter months. When individuals complain of increased symptoms during winter months it may be that the estrogen/progesterone levels have fallen excessively much like at the end of the monthly cycle. If increased symptoms occur in spring it may be an over abundance of estrogen/progesterone or a ratio variation between estrogen/progesterone.

In one study, progesterone levels were found not to change throughout the month in CPP individuals. There was a significantly higher incidence of galactorrhea (milky discharge of breasts), polycystic ovaries, endometriosis, uterine fibroids, and ovarian cysts. This imbalance may result in higher than normal levels of progesterone in relation to estrogen during the first part of the cycle and lower than normal progesterone in relation to estrogen levels the second 14 days. This imbalance could cause chronic immune system activation and eventually immune system fatigue and dysfunction.

When the ratio of estrogen to progesterone is abnormal the potential for sleep disturbance, fatigue, muscle pain, depression and confusion can increase. As estrogen is relatively lower calcium absorption drops leading to muscle pain and fatigue. Thyroid hormone T4 conversion to T3 drops which leads to metabolism abnormalities at the cellular level. Fatigue, sluggishness, hunger, and feeling cold are symptoms of dysfunctional metabolism. Decreased circulation to the brain, decreased potentiation of serotonin and enkephalins in the brain can lead to mental confusion, depression, and memory problems.

The ratio of estrogen/progesterone to testosterone levels is another consideration in CPP symptoms. Testosterone, the male adrogen, facilitates muscle definition and strength and the distribution of fat around the waistline. An imbalance in the ratio of estrogen/progesterone to testosterone can aggravate muscle spasms and increase pain perception.

Relaxin is a little known hormone present in both female and males that may also affect CPP symptoms. Relaxin is produced in the ovaries, uterus and breast tissues in the female. In the male it is produced in the seminal tubule. Relaxin levels vary throughout the month in females in conjunction with the estrogen/progesterone cycle. It is usually measurable in the blood stream seven to ten days after ovulation in females. It is difficult to measure in males. During pregnancy relaxin is present at levels ten time higher than in the non-pregnant state. It is the third major pregnancy hormone, estrogen and progesterone being the other two. Relaxin affects the production, elasticity and remodeling of collagen which is a major component in muscle, ligaments and tendons. Relaxin, through its affects on collagen synthesis and remodeling, causes ligaments and connective tissues to elongate and relax. It also affects the smooth muscle tone of blood vessels, increasing dilation of vessels.

Post-Traumatic Stress Disorder

Post-Traumatic Stress Disorder (PTSD) and Chronic Pelvic Pain are often seen in conjunction with each other in an individual. While the assessment procedures may be the same for any CPP individual, the methods, techniques and interpersonal communications used during treatment will be different in someone with PTSD.

Incidence

In the U.S. sexual and physical abuse is the number one reason for injury in the female population, and is one of the primary reasons for PTSD. Studies indicate the incidence of abuse is between 20%-50% in adult women. Abused women experience a higher frequency of functional diagnosis and somatic complaints in contrast to organic diagnosis and physical complaints. Childhood sexual abuse and/or physical abuse is closely related to chronic pain and pelvic pain in adulthood. The risk of chronic pain doubles in women who have experienced abuse. Walker et. al. found women with chronic pelvic pain had significantly higher prevalence of sexual abuse than the non pain control group. In another study he found an 86% predictive value of childhood sexual abuse in the CPP population compared to chronic pain in other areas of the body. It is estimated that one in three girls and one in seven boys are abused before the age of eighteen. Women reported abuse ten times more than men. Sexual abuse is fifteen percent of all reported child abuse. It is most common to experience a combination of physical, sexual, and emotional abuse.

Seventy eight percent of individuals who have experienced sexual abuse reported bladder incontinence in a study by Bernier. Douglas et. al. found sexual and physical abuse was prevalent in women diagnosed with gastrointestinal disorders and pelvic pain. Constipation is significantly increased in women who have experienced sexual abuse compared to those that have not. Forty-four percent reported previous sexual or physical abuse. Abused patients were more likely than non-abused patients to report pelvic pain.

In spite of the correlations found, it is important that the clinician not assume an individual who comes for treatment has experienced abuse.

Perpetrator

Children are most often abused by someone they know. A father, step father, uncle, brother, grandparent, neighbor, family friend, baby-sitter, teacher, aunt, or mother are some examples. The most common abuser is the heterosexual male. Females perpetrate the abuse in 4-44% of the cases depending on the setting. For instance in a day care setting the abuser is female 40-50% of the time. Females are often more covert abusers with the abuse being more subtle and seductive disguised in the form of caretaking and nurturing behaviors.

Psychosocial Impact

The presence of childhood sexual and physical abuse in women with pelvic pain makes it important to assess psychosocial aspects as well as physical aspects during a complete evaluation. Incidence of lifetime depression is five times greater in pelvic pain individuals than in the non-pain population. The more an individual perceives locus of control as being outside of herself the greater is the frequency and severity of depression and pelvic pain.

The impact in daily life is significant, they describe an underlying "dis ease" with life. The extremes are often obvious in their lives. Self care, moderation and homeostasis are not present. They often view chaos as a valuable tool to keep "dis ease" at bay. Smooth sailing for a period of time will nearly always be actively disrupted by one crisis or another. Symptoms can include low self esteem, secrecy, compulsions, addictions, self mutilation, fears, phobias, panic attacks, shame, self hate, rage, perfectionism, control, inhibited or exaggerated sexuality, and flashbacks. Coping strategies utilized to survive include minimizing, rationalizing, denying, forgetting, splitting, controlling, chaos, hyper-alertness, comedic humor, busyness, fantasizing, mental illness, eating disorders, lying, stealing, gambling, religion, and extreme sexual behavior.

Physical Impact

The physical aspects of CPP secondary to sexual or physical abuse are important to attend to in assessment and treatment. There can be trigger points, tender points, scar tissue, muscle holding patterns, or muscle spasms resulting from the physical trauma of the abuse. In addition, the physiological changes that occur alter the function of every system in the body. Muscle resting tone is elevated, and breathing patterns are altered to reflect the hyperalert status of the abuse prone life. Heart rate and blood pressure often become chronically elevated. Every organ system is altered. These changes are relatively hidden from the public eye. The physical injury aspect of sexual abuse is not obvious like a broken leg would be. Yet, every minute of the day the individual is coping with the aftermath.

"Doctor-Patient" Relationship

An individual who has experienced abuse has been robbed of the ability to trust. It is therefore very difficult to trust a heath care provider. In some cases that distrust extends to being in the same room alone with the "doctor". The individual, if abused as a child, has not developed the ability to provide for her own needs in a healthy way. Following through on a home program may be impossible alone. The urge to please is dominant so lying about daily activities occurs frequently. It is very difficult for the individual to set boundaries or limits. Shame, secrecy, and dissociation from her body are predominant so it is difficult to accurately inform a health care professional as to what the true symptoms are and how her needs can best be met. Part of her body has been incredibly hurt yet it is not visible to anyone. There is often denial that abuse ever happened which leads to physiological numbing and disconnection of that body part from the brain. Over time a separation of body information from the head brain occurs. The longer the time frame of secrecy, the more involved the dissociation becomes.

Creating an Environment Where Sexual and Physical Abuse Can Be Discussed

An abused client needs the safety of a private, comfortable, quiet room. The clinician needs to stay in the room rather than going in and out seeing more than one person at a time. It is important to give them your undivided attention if at all possible. The client needs to remain in the same room for evaluation and treatment.

During the initial history and first visit the client is fully dressed and seated in a comfortable chair, not poised on a treatment table dressed in a paper gown. The client may need to have a support person during the first one or two visits. They should not be left alone to wait in a small room alone for any length of time.

Assessment Tools and Techniques

In order to obtain accurate information, open ended questions and non-judgemental listening are two important assessment techniques. Questions that encourage factual and feeling responses rather than yes or no answers are best. Non-judgemental listening involves the clinician maintaining an open, accepting body posture, sincere eye contact, accepting nods and verbage. These are all ways of validating the client's experience.

During the history taking be alert to hints from the client that he/she may have been abused. If the client says she wasn't abused but you suspect she was, ask again later. Recognize symptoms of sexual abuse in body language, verbage and facts given during the history. If the client brings up abuse once, then stops talking about it, bring it up again later. Do not ignore the topic of sexual abuse, don't be afraid of it. If the client discloses abuse, ask questions like "when did it occur," "how does it effect you now?" Check for drug or alcohol problems. Ask if the client has or is receiving counseling for the abuse. The client is the expert about his/her abuse experience. Believe the story and don't minimize abuse and its effect. Affirming any statement of feelings he/she expresses, is essential.

Observe body language to see if it coincides with the description of the problem. The conscious brain may not have access to the information but the physical body does.

Have the individual draw and describe what she feels in each part of the body. What areas are blank? How does she draw in the body diagram? Is each part hot, cold, what is the color, texture? This can help determine dissociation behavior which is separating from a part of the body that holds memories of abuse.

Assess the duration and intensity of the individual's work and physical activity or exercise. Determine the reasons for each activity in her daily life. Is it for pleasure, stress relief, weight control, habit? Determine nutritional status, fluid consumption, caffeine, typical daily meals.

When touching, palpating, or moving body parts during assessment, always obtain permission before touching and direct attention to the body part that is to be moved or touched. Help the individual remain connected to her body. If you notice a sense of being far away, stop what you are doing and inquire gently about what is happening. Feel and watch body language as you do any testing. Before doing any resistive strength testing or repetitive movement testing be sure to know the individual's ability to give accurate information and limit the assessment appropriate to the ability.

While taking the history observe facial expressions, body language, and age appropriate words and tone of voice. An individual with a sexual abuse history may switch into childlike behavior for periods of time. Observe appearance for extremes of dress, perfume, etc. The individual may exaggerate the feminine side or try to deny it with slovenly or manly attire.

The first one or two visits are a time to develop trust and safety for the individual and a time for the clinician to understand her needs. At the end of the assessment it is important to clearly delineate the therapist-client roles and boundaries as well as mutual goals to be worked toward.

SECTION FOUR

What is Effective
Medical Management and Self Care?

Chapter 14

Medical Specialists
and Medications

A physician who knows about CPP is the keystone of an effective team which also includes the individual, family members, other medical and complementary care personnel, friends, relatives, and work acquaintances. Most frequently the physician is an internist, family practice physician, neurologist, obstetrician/gynecologist, urologist or gastroenterologist. Essential aspects of a health care team are: knowledge, interest, and the concept of a self-care model for chronic pain.

The physician will take a complete history of present and past problems. He/she will review the results of blood tests and X-rays as well as the results of special tests used to eliminate other illnesses which could be causing the same symptoms. The physician will also perform a physical exam. The diagnosis of CPP is made after evaluation of all these factors.

Once a diagnosis is made, the physician recommends appropriate medications, follows up on the patient's response to treatment and evaluates any side effects. The physician coordinates the health care team in developing treatment strategies, including techniques for pain relief, sleep disturbance relief, daily self-care management, self-care crisis management, and quality of life restoration working toward a return to work and full function. The physician's ultimate role is to assist the individual in taking control of his/her illness, teaching self-care techniques for pain, fatigue, and other symptoms. The physician assists the individual in knowing when and how the medical team can be helpful.

Obstetrician-Gynecologist

Abdominal and pelvic pain are the predominant symptoms for CPP individuals. An obstetrician/ gynecologist (Ob/Gyn) is involved in differentiating the symptoms of tumors and infections of the reproductive organs and intestines from CPP. An Ob/Gyn recommends medication and performs surgical procedures to alleviate symptoms of CPP. During pregnancy, the biomechanical and hormonal changes may increase CPP. When the obstetrician is aware that CPP is a factor, care can be specialized to provide for optimum comfort and function. Obstetricians prescribe pessaries and vaginal dilators.

Urologist

Urologists diagnose and treat bladder problems. Since CPP affects smooth muscle and circulation in the bladder, symptoms of urgency, frequency, enuresis (uncontrolled leaking of urine), lower abdominal discomfort and flank or kidney pain in the absence of test findings of infection, obstruction or tumors are often linked to CPP. Interstitial cystitis includes symptoms of frequent urination (multiple times an hour during the day and more than two times at night), feeling the urge to urinate but having very little flow and a bloated feeling of discomfort/ pain in the lower abdomen. Urethral syndrome symptoms (frequent urination and discomfort with urination) can be caused by CPP or fibromyalgia. CPP can be involved in stress, urge, mixed and enuresis types of incontinence. Since CPP symptoms include bladder and bowel symptoms, the effective treatment of urologic problems often significantly reduces the CPP symptoms or vice versa. Urologists perform special tests and surgical procedures for the specific bladder conditions.

Gastroenterologist

A gastroenterologist deals with disorders of the gastrointestinal tract including complaints of abdominal pain, constipation, rectal or tailbone pain. Tests done include anorectal manometry and colon transit. Anorectal manometry is a test to look at rectal sensation and internal and external sphincter function. Colon transit studies look at mouth to anus transit time of food.

Other tests include a flexible sigmoidoscopy, a test to look at conditions of the colon using a lighted tube; a colonoscopy or a barium enema, a test to look at possible pathologies followed by an x-ray, dependent on the severity of the pain and symptoms.

A general or colorectal surgeon will perform surgical procedures of the gastrointestinal tract.

Orthopedic Surgeon

An orthopedist is a surgeon who operates on bones and joints and is an expert in LBP. When multiple symptoms coexist with the core CPP symptoms many individuals look for more than one diagnosis. Symptoms such as numbness and tingling or shooting pain can bring about concern that other problems such as tendinitis, bursitis, or nerve compression, may be playing a role. Because CPP can be associated with all these myriad symptoms it is advisable to treat the CPP first and see how well the other symptoms respond. Many times the other problems are resolved with general CPP treatment. An orthopedic surgeon is consulted if unusual symptoms persist. An orthopedic surgeon who is familiar with CPP and LBP will ask the key questions, evaluate, and treat for the specific orthopedic problem. Treatments include medications and surgical procedures.

Neurologist

A neurologist evaluates and treats dysfunction of the nervous system. Diagnostic tests are performed to rule out diseases of the nervous system such as multiple sclerosis, Parkinson's disease or amyotrophic lateral sclerosis. A neurologist performs nerve conduction velocity tests to determine if the pain, numbness, and tingling the individual describes is a nerve compression or transmission problem.

Where there is a second diagnosis in conjunction with CPP and LBP, treating both diagnoses simultaneously is the most effective approach. Any physician an individual chooses should have a working knowledge of CPP and its implications.

As one individual said about finding a doctor. "I have looked long and hard for my doctor. The one I have now listens, always gives me options for treatment, involves my family, and encourages me to be independent and try new things. He is wonderful about keeping up on new medications that might help."

Naturopathic Medicine

Naturopathic medicine focuses on facilitating the body's innate healing abilities. Natural medicines support the body and work in conjunction with the immune system to restore health. Naturopathic medicine addresses the physical, mental, and emotional aspects of dysfunction. Treatment possibilities include nutritional analysis, dietary alterations, constitutional homeopathic remedies, botanical medicines, hormone therapy, counseling and hydrotherapy. Nutritional analysis includes food intake, digestive capacity, and elimination patterns. Dietary recommendations may include foods to avoid such as coffee, chocolate, vinegar, pickled foods, acidic plant foods, alcohol, carbonated drinks, shellfish, white sugar, white flour, artificial additives and preservatives, and processed foods. A detoxification diet is often recommended. Supplementation can include omega 3 and 6 fatty acids and multiple vitamins. Constitutional homeopathy can include an individually prescribed remedy to address symptoms and susceptibility of the immune system. Botanical medicines are used to affect inflammation, liver function, the digestive system, nervous system, endocrine and circulatory systems. Hormone therapy can include DHEA, melatonin and phytoestrogen and progesterone. Hydrotherapy includes herbal, Epsom salts, and mineral baths.

Medications

Chronic pelvic pain can be treated medically with the concept that long-term pain is an illness in itself. Other disease specific diagnoses should be treated appropriately as separate entities. These diagnoses may involve bladder, bowel or uterine pathology. Since the severity of CPP is not usually proportional to specifically identified tissue trauma effective medications are often directed at modulating pain through central as well as peripheral mechanisms. Goals in relation to medication effectiveness include: 1) relieve suffering, 2) restore sleep patterns, 3) restore daily activities and 4) improve quality of life.

Medications for Chronic Pelvic Pain
Peripheral Analgesics

Nonsteroidal Anti-Inflammatories – (NSAIDs)

Function:	Inhibits prostaglandin synthesis
Effect:	Blocks pain and inflammation at local tissue level
Dose:	600-800 mg/day for analgesic level
Side Effects:	Nausea, stomach pain, ulcers, fluid retention, renal toxicity in older individuals
Examples:	ibuprofen (Motrin, Advil), naproxen (Naprosyn, Aleve)

Adjuncts

Tricyclic Antidepressants (TCA)

Function:	Increase CNS neurotransmitter levels (serotonin and/or norepinephrine)
Effect:	Sedation, diminish fatigue, decrease pain, elevate mood
Dose:	5-75 mg often at bedtime - dose varies with drug
Side Effects:	Racing heart, nightmares, dizziness, tiredness, dry mouth, urinary retention, constipation, weight gain
Examples:	amitriptyline (Elavil) nortriptyline (Pamelor) doxepin (Sinequan) desipramine (Norpramin)

Cyclobenzaprine (Flexeril)
A tricyclic amine, it is a muscle relaxant.
10-40mg/day

Zolpidem (Ambien)
Function: Non-benzodiazepine sedative/hypnotic
Effect: Increased duration of sleep, decreased time to
              get to sleep
Dose: 5-10 mg
Side Effects: Memory problems, daytime drowsiness, dizziness,
              headache, nausea
Note: Short term treatment of insomnia only, 7-10 days,
              minimal dependency/addictive qualities

Serotonin Reuptake Inhibitors
Function: Blocks destruction of serotonin so its effects last longer
              (controls food intake, temperature regulation, anxiety)
Effect: Diminish pain, fatigue, and anxiety; improve mood
Dose: 20-200mg depending on agent
Side Effects: Anxiety, nervousness, insomnia, tremor, dizziness,
              libido changes
Examples: fluoxetine (Prozac)
              sertraline (Zoloft)
              paroxetine (Paxil)
              venafaxine (Effexor)

Nefazadone (Serzone)
Function: Inhibits uptake of serotonin and norepinephrine
Effect: Decrease pain, diminish fatigue
Side Effects: Nausea, headaches, postural hypotension
Note: Not to be taken with monoamine oxidase inhibitors

Central Acting Opiod Analgesics
Function: Binds to opiate receptors in brain to alter
              brain perception.
Effect: Decrease pain and anxiety, improve sleep
Dose: Varies with agent
Side Effects: Drowsiness, decreased physical activity, mood changes,
              respiratory depression, mental slowness, dizziness

Examples: methodone (Dolophine), morphine, butorphanol \
(Stadol), fentanyl (Duragesic), hydrocodone (Vicodin,
Lortab), meperidine (Demerol), morphine, oxycodone
(Percodan, Percocet, Oxycontin), propoxyphene
(Darvocet)

Tramadol (Ultram)

Function: Increases serotonin and norepinephrine, bonds to
opiate receptors; a synthetic analgesic
Effect: Inhibits pain perception, decreases pain
Dose: 50 mg, 2-4/day
Side Effects: Dizziness, nausea, constipation, headaches, postural
hypotension
Note: Minimal dependency/addictive qualities

Antibiotics

Appropriate if chronic infections such as Pelvic Inflammatory Disease (PID), possible subacute genital tract infection, chronic urethral syndrome, or bladder infection is present.

Estrogen/Progesterone

Appropriate if female is over 40 and/or perimenopausal. Incontinence, irritation and inflammation of the vagina or urethra can be significantly improved using phytoestrogen or animal estrogen/ progesterone. The estrogen/progesterone can be taken orally, by injection, patch, or cream.

Combination Therapies

- **Prozac** and **Sinequan**
  Restlessness caused by Prozac balanced by Sinequan quieting
- **Prozac** and **Elavil**
  Elavil at night restores normal sleep pattern and Prozac in the morning helps decrease morning drowsiness.
- **Opiates** and **NSAIDS**

Note: Any sedating antidepressant at bedtime may be used with any of the SSRIs in the morning, for example trazadone (Desyrel), a sedative, used with sertraline (Zoloft), an SSRI.

Medication for Bladder Incontinence

Stress Incontinence

Generic Name	Brand Name
Ephedrine	Ephedrine
Pseudoephedrine	Sudafed
Phenylpropanolamine	Dexatrim
Imiprimine	Tofranil

These medications increase tone of the bladder outlet/internal urethral sphincter to prevent leaking.

Urge Incontinence

Generic Name	Brand Name
Propantheline	Pro-Banthine
Flavoxate	Urispas
Dicyclomine hydrochloride	Bentyl
Imiprimine	Tofranil
Oxybutynin	Ditropan, Ditropan XL
Hysoscyamine	Levsin
Tolterodine tartrate	Detrol

These medications decrease bladder contractions when the bladder tends to be overactive.

Medications for Bowel Incontinence

Irritable Bowel Syndrome

Generic Name	Brand Name
Hysoscyamine	Bentyl,
Dicyclomine hydrochloride	Levsin
Tricyclic antidepressants	
Amitriptyline	Elavil
Nortriptyline	Pamelor
	Imodium

Some individuals experience side effects from the medications used to treat incontinence. The side effects can be minor and last only a few days after initiation of the medication. If they significantly change the individual's behavior or ability to function or if the symptoms continue longer it is important to contact the prescribing physician and describe the problem. Often a change in dosage or a change in medication is

Chapter 14: Medical Specialists and Medications

possible. Side effects of incontinence medication can include dry mouth, dizziness, headaches, mental confusion, anxiety, nervousness, blurred vision, extremity weakness, joint or muscle pain, constipation or diarrhea, lethargy, somnolence, and insomnia.

Trigger Point Injections

Trigger points, when pressure is applied, are painful at the site and refer pain to other areas of the body. They are a sign of a myofascial pain pattern or syndrome. Tender points are exquisitely painful at the site of pressure only.

Injections into trigger points in CPP are appropriate if there is myofascial pain. The trigger points are injected with:

- Saline solution
- Lidocaine, procaine (local anesthetics)
- Cortisone – in small amounts, less frequently. There may be increased pain for up to 48 hours after the injection, then there should be a decrease in pain over the long term. Systemic side effects almost never occur if the volume injected is below 5 cc, but this is dependent on the potency of the steroid.

Herbal / Natural Products

- Licorice – Use natural not synthetic form. Used to increase blood volume and increase blood pressure in vasopressor syncope.
- Melatonin – Secreted by pineal gland and made from serotonin. It helps set the sleep/wake cycle.
- Valerian – Used to treat sleep disturbance.
- Echinacea – Used to decrease pain.
- Calms Forte – Used to improve sleep and anxiety.
- Rhus Toxicodendron – Used to treat stiffness.
- Ginger – Used to improve irritable bowel syndrome.
- Cayenne – Used to improve circulation and digestion, to decrease pain.
- Peppermint – Used to improve digestion and decrease intestinal cramping.
- Chamomile – Used to improve sleep and decrease intestinal cramping.

Note: herbals are not FDA controlled.

Chapter 15

General Self Care Management

Self Care Stabilizing Loops

The knowledge from your Personal Assessment in Chapter 11 & 13 enables you to begin managing your CPP more effectively. The goal of any individual with CPP symptoms is to function well and fully in daily life, work, social, recreational, and family activities with pain-free energy. This goal, at the physiological level, requires efficient and effective muscle work and rest cycles. Muscles of the arms, legs, back, abdomen and neck – the voluntary muscles – must function efficiently and effectively. Additionally, smooth muscles of the heart, lungs, gut, bladder and reproductive organs that are controlled by the autonomic nervous system must function efficiently to accomplish pain-free daily activities. To optimize the function of muscles it is necessary for them to receive and absorb the essential nutrients and oxygen needed for energy production (metabolism) within their cell structures and to effectively eliminate the waste products left after the metabolic process is completed. The goal is to achieve normal function in daily and work activities, in leisure time activities, and during sleep.

Treatment

Ideally the individual is working with a health care professional to set goals and monitor progress of each treatment approach. It is important to find a trusted and interested professional to be your coach and guide the recovery process. Treatment can include medication and self-care. No pill, surgery, or counseling has proven to be a cure. Medications can help but in most cases medication does not completely alleviate the symptoms over the long term. Self care becomes the primary treatment to alleviate the symptoms of CPP and optimize functional and work activities.

It is common for an individual with CPP to comment, "I am too busy with my family and work to do all that self care stuff," or "I did the self care routine for several months and got better but it didn't last when I went back to my usual routine," or "My family (spouse) thinks I am being selfish and self centered when I spend so much time on me." With these comments it is no wonder that the best treatment is often ignored.

Self care is a form of work, a job that must come first if the individual is to function optimally in the home, family and work place. It is a job that must be maintained over the life time. The individual brushes her teeth and washes her face every day as a given part of life. The self care routine for CPP is the same as brushing and washing. It is forever and important. The individual with CPP deserves to include those self care items that provide health and enable her/him to function in a healthy way with family and society.

Sometimes the individual is able to gradually integrate the self care routine into life activities without changing the daily routine much. Other times it is necessary to interrupt the normal routine for a time and emphasize self care to realize what being a healthy person can feel like. Then family, social and work activities are gradually added back in when the self care routine is effectively in place. It is important that the self care routine remain at the core of daily life. It is not an add on when there is time.

Case Study

Mary tells of using self care techniques in a concentrated way for six weeks and feeling a lot better, sleeping, exercising, using Physiological Quieting, and changing her nutritional patterns. Then her physician told her she could go back to work. Her family said they were glad she was well now and could start doing what she did before. Her co-workers welcomed her back and she returned to her same job. Within two weeks she was exhausted, aching and painful and expressed confusion and frustration about what to do now.

The answer to the scenario described above is continual self care.

Self care is the best solution to a chronic problem. It needs to be a deserved priority on a daily basis. There will still be ups and downs but the windows of "feeling good" will be larger and the crisis times will be less intense.

To discover the best self care approach for each individual takes time and exploration. Each individual will be unique in his/her needs in spite of similarities throughout the population as a whole.

When a new technique like exercise is started, it is important to start slowly and gradually increase the intensity and repetitions. As with any other sensory input, the CPP nervous system over-responds to the sensation and action of new events. That can exhaust the body and mind quickly or set off the teeter-totter imbalance within the many body systems. Floating through exercises, doing a few repetitions of each exercise, and emphasizing rest as much as work is the basic rule for all new endeavors. Work and recreational related activities must be approached the same way. Constantly quieting the systems keeps the balance and prevents increased pain, fatigue and dysfunction.

To get started on your program of healthy living remember you were created as a deserving human being and your most important job is to care for your body and mind in the ways it needs to be healthy. There cannot be a separation between the body and mind, the body is equal to the mind in value, intelligence and work capabilities and deservedness.

The General CPP Self Care Stabilizing Loop

The General Self Stabilizing Loop includes the self care spiral.
(Figure 30)

- Sleep Routine
- Physiological Quieting
- Nutrition
- Exercise
- Medication
- Acupressure/Massage

- Positive Self Talk
- Rest/Work Cycles
- Pacing/Prioritizing
- Modalities
- Journaling

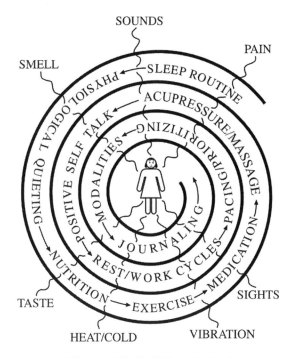

Figure 30: Self Care Spiral

The General Chronic Pelvic Pain Self Care Stabilizing Loop items are listed in order of priority. Sleep protocol, Physiological Quieting, and nutrition are combined in the first step. It may take up to a month to incorporate these new behaviors. No one can expect to turn over a new leaf in a day or a week. Persevering along a path of small steps and positive actions will result in decreased symptoms. Check off the items as you progress through the First Step Protocol. (Figure 31)

General CPP Self Care Stabilizing Loop

	M	T	W	T	F	S	S	Comments
First Step Protocol								
Sleep								
Defined bedtime/rise time								
8-9 hours/sleep								
snack at bedtime								
remove caffeine								
PQ at bedtime								
appropriate bed clothing and pillows								
environmental stimuli stabilized								
Physiological Quieting								
listen to PQ tape at night								
hourly PQ for 30 seconds								
Nutrition								
reduce/eliminate								
simple sugars								
caffeine								
alcohol								
6-8 glasses water daily								
vitamin / mineral food / supplements								
amino acid foods/supplements								
reduce/eliminate detrimental foods								
Second Step Protocol								
Exercise -								
Roll In & Out								
20-30 min. daily Aerobic								
Medication								
1.								
2.								
Massage								
Positive Self Talk								
1.								
2.								
Rest/Work Cycles								
Pacing/Prioritize								
Dress								
Modalities								
Journaling								

Figure 31: General Self Care Stabilizing Loop

Sleep Protocol

Sleep is the most important first step in health for individuals with chronic pelvic pain. Deep sleep occurs when there is replacement and repair of all cells of body and mind. During sleep it is important that your body systems remain relatively stable. For example:

- your temperature needs to remain relatively stable,
- your blood sugar needs to remain relatively stable,
- your muscle tension/tightness needs to remain relatively relaxed,
- your mind activity needs to remain relatively quiet,
- your oxygen levels need to remain relatively stable.

To that end self care techniques that help these systems remain stable will be the first ones to learn and integrate into daily life. These include:

- Physiological Quieting (PQ) – breathing, hand warming, and PQ audiotape
- Eliminate nutritional stimulants – caffeine, alcohol
- Minimize environmental irritants – noise, odor, temperature, light
- Schedule regular and adequate time for sleep.

As these become regular habits in daily life, pain, fatigue, and associated symptoms can significantly decrease.

Since restful sleep is a top priority for CPP individuals, planning an individual routine for sleep is important. "I want to be able to get to sleep, sleep through the night without pain and frequent waking. I want to feel rested and limber when I awake," Jody tells her health care consultant.

To get to sleep:

- Remove stimulants such as caffeine from your diet. This includes any coffee, tea, soda or chocolate that contains caffeine. Some headache and pain remedies contain caffeine and should be changed to another non-caffeine containing medication. Caffeine is a stimulant to the ANS, increasing pain perception, stimulating the brain's arousal systems and facilitating wakefulness. It is also a bladder irritant so it can increase the times you need to go to the bathroom at night.
- Hunger and/or hypoglycemia can increase insomnia symptoms so eating a light carbohydrate snack like a piece of whole wheat toast

or a banana along with a small amount of a milk product or protein just before bedtime can improve sleep. Milk products contain tryptophan, a natural chemical that has a calming and relaxing effect on the nervous system and is a precursor to serotonin. Milk products also contain calcium which helps with sleep and muscle relaxation. Carbohydrates help speed tryptophan to the brain.

- A regular bedtime and wake up time is important for individuals with sleep disturbance. Eight to ten hours of sleep each night is important. Growth hormone in CPP individuals is produced in greatest amounts during the early morning hours, so the best sleep for CPP is sometimes termed "sleeping in" by others. Growth hormone is essential for the growth and repair of all body cells. Shift changes at a job are not conducive to health with CPP individuals since the body clock needs to practice the same routine over a long period of time and is hypersensitive to disruption.

- The hour before bedtime needs to be a time of winding down, a time for yourself and quiet enjoyment. It is not a time to be balancing the checkbook, paying the bills, or settling a family disagreement. Instead, try soft music, a hot bath, a good book, or writing in a journal. This is the time to use Physiological Quieting in preparation for sleep.

To stay asleep:

- Use a supportive mattress that has its own soft pad or place an egg crate mattress under the sheet and mattress pad. Try different pillows until you find the best one for your head and neck, one that is most comfortable through the night and enables you to wake up with minimal feelings of stiffness and soreness in your neck and shoulders. Use a pillow between your knees and hug one when you sleep on your side. When sleeping on your back, place pillows under your knees as well as supporting your head and neck. You may even want pillows to support each shoulder and arm. Sleeping on your stomach is not recommended because of the extreme position it puts your neck and low back.

- Wear warm night wear with long sleeves and long pants. Some people even wear socks, gloves and nightcaps to help maintain body temperature while sleeping.

- Warm the bed before you get in using a heating pad or electric mattress pad. Turn it off before you go to sleep.
- Eliminate environmental factors that can arouse a light sleeper. Dark out shades and a sleep mask keep out light. A sound conditioner which produces white noise or ear plugs block out the background noise of car engines, horns, and people talking. Essential oils such as lavender and eucalyptus can facilitate restfulness and block out other stimulating smells. Stabilize the room heat so the temperature is the same all night and use blankets which are adequate for the duration of sleep.
- Exercise moderately 20-30 minutes some time during the day at least three hours before bedtime. Exercising in the evening stimulates the nervous system and may increase alertness and wakefulness.
- If you wake up during the night move to a comfortable position, then relax muscles head to toe into the bed and begin diaphragmatic breathing, hand warming, and positive self statements. Know that your body and mind are in a restful state even if you do not perceive that you are asleep.
- If you can't get back to sleep after a half an hour to an hour get up, read a book, write in a journal, or do some gentle exercise, and then try to sleep again later.
- Use prescribed medication consistently. Consult a physician about changes in sleep patterns.

The goal: **sleep through the night, wake rested and limber!**

Physiological Quieting™

An individual responds to events in daily life through chemical changes within the body and brain. The alarm in the morning is perceived by the ear, transferred to the brain center for hearing by chemical events within the nerve, then interpreted by the head and gut control centers which send messages to the rest of the body through additional chemicals saying, "open your eyes, jump out of bed, get dressed." Chemical messages are different depending on how the event is perceived by the head and gut brain. If the event is perceived as an emergency, a fight or flight event, chemicals such as adrenaline and testosterone are released in increased amounts; if the event is perceived as a normal, easy life event by the brain and body the chemicals released are different and give activating but calmer directions to all organs and tissues.

CPP individuals' brain centers and nervous systems tend to respond to life events with excessive fight or flight chemicals rather than quieting chemicals. The autonomic nervous system that controls heart rate, breathing, stomach and intestine activity, bladder function, and circulation tends to send out more fight or flight chemicals than quieting chemicals. We say it has a high idle at rest, always ready to jump. The on/off switch for full activation is hypersensitive. This means even normal daily events may activate chemical messengers that are meant for use only during short periods of high stress. This constant activation of stress chemicals is destructive to the body over the long term. Circulation to muscles is decreased so muscles ache from lack of oxygen and accumulation of waste products. Breathing rate increases and breathing is shallow and irregular so the CPP individual complains of shortness of breath and low endurance during aerobic activity. Heart rate increases and is often irregular, chest pain and pressure are experienced. Stomach and intestinal activity increases. Excessive abnormal smooth muscle contractions can cause stomach and abdominal pain, diarrhea, and indigestion. Light, irregular sleep can prevent repair and replacement of body cells.

It is important to use management techniques that quiet the high idle or high resting level of the nervous system. It is important to use management techniques that assist the autonomic nervous system in responding to daily events with "calm" chemical messengers to organ systems instead of "fight or flight" chemical messengers.

These techniques are termed Physiological Quieting™. Physiological Quieting™ (PQ) is an integral part of a successful CPP management system. Its goals are:

- to rebalance the ANS regulation of circulation and internal organ function (heart, lungs, intestines),
- to normalize the release of chemical messengers from the head and gut control centers to the rest of the body, and
- to equalize the feedback message loop from the body to the head compared to the message loop from the head to the body telling it what to do, what it needs for health and well being.

The divisions of the ANS are the sympathetic, the parasympathetic, and the enteric (gut). The ANS directs/regulates the activity of all organs of the body. When this "body-brain" feedback loop is balanced, the individual is in a state of health. When the body-brain feedback loop is unbalanced, the individual is in a state of dis-ease. It is important to balance the body messages with the head messages, to balance the sympathetic (fight or flight) messages with the parasympathetic (quieting) messages, and the gut (enteric) messages with the head (CNS) messages to have optimal health for CPP individuals. An overactive sympathetic nervous system leads to decreased circulation, increased muscle resting tone (both smooth and striated), and myofascial tissue thickening (Figure 32) which results in pain, fatigue, and limitations of daily activities.

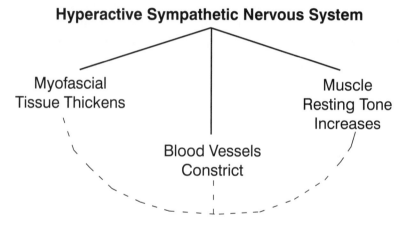

Figure 32: Hyperactive Sympathetic Nervous System

With a well balanced ANS and with smooth running feedback loops between body and brain, sleep improves, muscle function improves, circulation improves, and pain and fatigue diminish. Physiological Quieting techniques are targeted to balance the ANS and its feedback loops with the CNS. The three major techniques in Physiological Quieting are:

- Breathing
- Hand Warming
- Body/Mind Quieting

Breathing

Some CPP individuals have a sense of dyspnea (air hunger) even in a resting state. During exercise an CPP individual's breathing pattern often is irregular when normal individuals would have extremely regular breathing. The diaphragm, the major breathing muscle, becomes dysfunctional much as other muscles do in CPP. Accessory breathing muscles in the neck and chest take over for the diaphragm. Breathing affects tissue oxygen levels, body metabolism, heart rate and the body's acid base balance. When breathing is erratic and the muscle action producing breathing patterns is changed, these physiological processes are severely altered. Heart rate is increased, nerve/muscle resting level is elevated, and blood pressure changes due to breathing changes. Symptoms described by CPP individuals that can be directly attributed to hyperventilation, the most drastic form of erratic breathing, include: shortness of breath, chest pain, choking or smothering sensation, dizziness, numbness and tingling in hands and feet, hot and cold flashes, faintness, trembling, and fear or anxiety feelings. With this in mind, returning to diaphragmatic breathing becomes an important aspect of CPP management.

Basic Exercise

The diaphragm is a large sheetlike muscle that rests in a dome shape in the chest from the nipple area to the bottom of the rib cage and the spine. As you inhale the dome flattens and pulls down to the bottom of the rib cage. During exhale the diaphragm moves back to the dome shape. When breathing correctly, the shoulder and chest areas remain quiet, the jaw is relaxed, and the teeth are separated. Inhale, 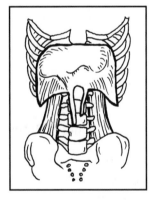 let your abdomen rise, exhale, let it fall. There is equal time for inhale and exhale. Inhaling through the nose, exhaling through the mouth or nose. Exhale is passive and quiet.

Diaphragmatic breathing eases and reverses the biochemical effects of hyperventilation and makes it easier for air to flow into the lungs. Practice diaphragmatic breathing initially in a reclined position, then in sitting and standing. Practice hourly during the day, 7-8 breaths.

Advanced Exercise

An advanced breathing exercise that helps to normalize diaphragm muscle function in relation to other body functions is the following:

- In a comfortable, supported position focus on low, slow diaphragmatic breathing.
- Now add: arch low back slightly with inhale, flatten low back with exhale.
- When this is easy add: roll legs out slightly with inhale, roll legs in with exhale.
- When this is easy add: roll palms up with inhale, roll palms down with exhale.
- When this is easy add: rock chin up slightly with inhale, rock chin down with exhale.

Practice 5-10 of these total body breaths in the morning before you get up and as you go to sleep at night.

Hand Warming

Circulation to muscles, nerves, internal organs, and the brain is often significantly decreased in CPP individuals. Some CPP individuals describe being core cold, not being able to warm up. Their hands and feet are cold, their buttocks feel cold, even their internal organs feel cold. Often a cold feeling is a cardinal sign of worsening CPP symptoms of muscle aching and fatigue within the next 6-8 hours.

Decreased circulation means blood vessel constriction. Blood vessel walls have three layers, one of which is muscular. The muscular layer is controlled by the sympathetic (fight or flight) nervous system. An active sympathetic system causes constriction of the blood vessel wall, a quieting sympathetic system causes dilation or relaxation of the blood vessel wall, allowing more blood flow. When more blood flows through the vessels there is increased heat from the increased blood volume which results in hands, feet and other body parts warming. This increases circulation to all muscles, bringing in food and oxygen and carrying away waste products so muscles can function with greater energy and less pain and fatigue.

Hand warming is a technique to increase blood volume to body parts. Mental imaging and frequently repeated thoughts transfer to nerve activity that quiets the sympathetic (fight or flight) nervous system activity resulting in dilation of blood vessels. To accomplish this:

- Visualize the warmest place your hands can be, holding a warm cup of hot chocolate, holding your hands over a camp fire or radiator, or slipping your hands and feet in the hot sand of a beach on a summer day.
- Think of the warmest color and surround your hands and wrists with that color. Let that color flow into your hands, deep into the palms, fingers, wrists while they get warmer and warmer.
- Focus your attention on your hands and say to yourself, "My hands are warmer and warmer, warmth is flowing into my hands, warmer and warmer."

To accomplish a resetting of the ANS, to slow the high idle, it is necessary to practice the techniques that quiet the sympathetic system frequently for short periods. The instructions are:

"Practice hourly for 30-60 seconds, wherever you are. No one will know you are doing it." Put colored dots up around your work and home or buy a watch that buzzes every hour to remind you. Then hourly do:

- 7-8 slow, low diaphragmatic breaths
- Release jaw, quiet shoulders quiet chest
- 7-8 repetitions of hand warming

Body/Mind Quieting

Balancing the ANS (body control centers) with the CNS (head control centers) helps all organs and muscles be their healthiest. The head is used to bossing the body around. It is not used to listening to what the body needs and has to say. Initially it will take conscious practice to reconnect the body to mind message system.

However, with practice it will become automatic for the feedback loop between the body to the head to be as strong as the head to the body (Figure 33).

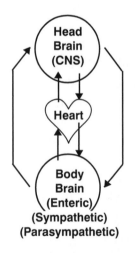

Figure 33: Body-Mind Feedback Loop

Body/mind quieting serves many important functions in helping CPP individuals. Excessive muscle resting levels and internal organ activity can be decreased through PQ of the body/mind. Abnormal sleep patterns are improved with PQ of the body/mind. Physiological Quieting of the body/mind assists the immune system in optimal functioning.

To accomplish body/mind quieting:

Find a quiet, warm room with a chair or bed that gives complete support from your head to your feet. Use pillows for support of your neck, low back, arms, and knees.

- Focus on your breathing, feel the pattern of breathing, let your abdomen rise with inhale, fall with exhale.
- Feel the warmth or coolness of your hands and feet, left side and right. Let your hands and feet feel warm, feel warmer and warmer.
- Feel the support of the bed or chair and release into that support, let your feet, legs, hips, back, shoulders, arms, neck and head sink deeper and deeper into that support.
- Focus on your face and neck. Notice where there is any tension or tightness, where there is quiet, calmness in each part of your face and neck muscles - your forehead, eyes, cheeks, tongue, throat, neck. Then say to yourself 3-4 times slowly, "My face and neck muscles are quiet and calm, my face and neck muscles are calmer and calmer."
- Proceed from head to toe in the same manner, focusing on head and neck, back (upper, middle and lower), shoulders and arms, hips and legs, chest and abdomen.
- Focus again on diaphragmatic breathing and hand warming.

One to two 20 minute body/mind quieting sessions a day are recommended. Try doing it 20 minutes before you get out of bed in the morning and 20 minutes before going to sleep at night using the Physiological Quieting audiotape.

Integrating Physiological Quieting throughout the day is an essential aspect of self care in CPP management.

Nutrition

The nutritional component in managing CPP can be controversial. Mary is told by her dietician to "eat a normal diet based on the food group pyramid." Jolene consults several traditional and alternative health care providers and uses nutritional supplements in addition to a balanced diet. The goal of good nutrition in CPP is to provide the needed food products that can be broken down and utilized for optimal body functions.

Nutrition is the next step in health for individuals with chronic pelvic pain. It comes before exercise because without adequate nutrition the muscle cells cannot function to perform exercise. The nutrients taken in through food and supplements are broken down and converted to usable substances by the digestive system. Considerations in healthy body use of nutritional components includes:

- adequate intake of needed nutrients
- elimination of detrimental nutrients
- adequate digestion of needed nutrients
- adequate absorption of needed nutrients
- adequate transportation of needed nutrients to body/ mind cells
- adequate metabolism of nutrients by cells for optimal cellular function

Adequate intake of needed nutrients can be different for each individual. There are general guidelines to begin with but it is trial and error to find out what works best for each individual's systems. General guidelines include:

- intake of water 6-8 glasses daily, 1 glass every 30 minutes of exercise
- regularly scheduled meals with balanced nutrient intake
- adequate vitamins, minerals, essential fatty acids, essential amino acids

Elimination of detrimental nutrients include:

- minimize caffeine – coffee, tea, chocolate, caffeinated soda
- minimize alcohol
- minimize sugar intake

Adequate digestion of needed nutrients is determined by the digestive system from the mouth to the rectum and anus. Considerations include:

- chewing ability in the mouth
- swallowing ability
- stomach digestion – breakdown of fruits
- small intestine digestion – breakdown of fats, carbohydrates
- colon function – absorption of water and nutrients
- rectum and anus – elimination of waste products

Individuals with CPP can complain of jaw/tooth pain which can change chewing habits. Chewing is the first step in digestion. Swallowing difficulties are common complaints in chronic pelvic pain. Choking and pain with swallowing affects what foods are eaten. Chest pain, stomach pain, and burping can be symptoms of stomach digestive problems. When stomach and small intestine digestion is affected, absorption of nutrients is a problem because the food is not being broken down adequately to enable its absorption into the blood stream. The same is true when the colon is dysfunctional. Irritable bowel syndrome is a common complaint of individuals with chronic pelvic pain. Alternating diarrhea and constipation can be from abnormal colon function which then affects the nutritional status of all cells of the body.

Certain foods, vitamins, or allergies to foods or chemicals do not cause chronic pelvic pain. Individuals may find specific foods that appear to exacerbate symptoms and others that appear to help. In general, any food or drink that is an irritant to the nervous system may exacerbate symptoms. For example, the caffeine in coffee, tea, soda and chocolate is a nervous system irritant and aggravates symptoms of muscle pain, sleep disturbance, and bladder irritability. On the other hand, food or drink that has a quieting affect may help decrease symptoms. For example, the high fiber in complex carbohydrates may quiet irritable bowel symptoms.

Adequate consumption of water and non-caffeinated fluids is important for an CPP individual's health. The increased accumulation of waste products in muscle and connective tissues increases pain. Adequate fluid consumption, 6-8 glasses per day, helps the circulatory system and kidneys process waste products.

CPP research reports decreased amounts of chemical messengers like serotonin and norepinephrine which are composed of amino acid chains. There are several ways to potentially increase the levels of these chemical messengers. These include:

- boost their production through vitamin and mineral supplements
- increase the consumption of protein
- add amino acids supplements to the diet.

No one vitamin, mineral or amino acid can function on its own. It takes a group process to accomplish the manufacture and distribution of the chemical messengers that regulate the body. The most important amino acids that help to form the chemical messengers include:

- L-tyrosine,
- L-phenylalanine, and
- L-tryptophan.

The precursor to serotonin is L-tryptophan. The precursors to norepinephrine are L-tyrosine and L-phenlyalanine. Vitamin B6 is especially important because it directs development of the chemical messenger necklaces of amino acids. Sugar is important to avoid because it competes with amino acids for absorption in the intestines. Increased sugar intake can result in decrease amino acid absorption for use in the chemical messengers' necklaces.

There are many kinds and brands of amino acids on the market. It is important to use the "free form" type of amino acid supplement so they are ready to be used by the body without complicated digestion processes. The pharmaceutical grade of amino acids is the desired grade. It can be taken in a powder or capsule.

Some CPP individuals try to eat pain and fatigue away. A common thought is, "If I just eat something I'll have more energy and not hurt as much." In other instances, when feelings of despair or depression are prevalent, the idea that food is a comforter leads to excessive calorie consumption. It is true that food can be quieting and comforting. Carbohydrates, for instance, tend to soothe the nervous system and gut. Yet it is important to recognize the symptoms and treat the pain, fatigue or depression, not try to cover them up or numb the senses with food.

It is vital to eat and drink adequately while exercising. Before starting an exercise program eat a light carbohydrate meal and drink 6-8 oz. of fluid. During workouts drink fluids every 10-15 minutes. It is important to consume a carbohydrate and protein meal within 15-20 minutes after exercise to replenish energy stores.

There are indications of decreased levels of magnesium in blood or muscle cells in some CPP individuals. Five to eight hundred milligrams of magnesium daily is recommended by some experts.

Vitamins and minerals that are important in a daily dietary plan for CPP include:

Vitamin C – 500 to 3000 mg/day
Vitamin B Complex – 25-50 mg/day
Calcium – 800-1000 mg/day for females premenopause,
       1200-1500 mg/day menopause or post menopause
       (300 mg = 8 oz. milk or 1 slice cheese)
Vitamin E – 200-400 IU/day
Vitamin D – 20 minutes of sunlight/day
Malic Acid – 1200-1400 mg/day
Magnesium – 500-800 mg/day
(See Vitamin/Mineral Chart on this page.)
Six to eight glasses of water daily! (decaffeinated fluids)

Vitamin/Mineral	Symptoms	Food Source
Vitamin B1	Fatigue Irritability Memory Loss Insomnia Muscle Weakness Numbness Tingling Headaches Increased Sensitivity to Pain Heart Palpitations	Wheat Germ Brewer's Yeast Soybeans Nuts Poultry Milk
Vitamin B5	Fatigue Muscle Weakness Muscle Cramps Hypoglycemia Constipation Diarrhea	Organ Meats Peanuts Wheat Germ Eggs Beans Peas

Vitamin/Mineral	Symptoms	Food Source
Vitamin B6	Irritability Insomnia Dizziness PMS Muscle Weakness Numbness Tingling Hair Loss Hypoglycemia	Brewer's Yeast Liver Salmon Nuts Brown Rice Meats Fish Soybeans
Vitamin B12	Mental Apathy Muscle Weakness Fatigue Depression Memory Loss Noise and Light Sensitivity Chest Pain	Liver Egg Yolk Sardines Salmon Crab
Vitamin C	Muscle Weakness Fatigue Confusion Joint Aches Bruising Poor Digestion Infections	Broccoli Brussel Sprouts Kale Parsley Green Peppers Rose Hips Lemons, Oranges. Tomatoes, Spinach, Cauliflower
Vitamin E	Muscle Pain Muscle Weakness PMS Decreased Circulation Infections Leg Pain Incoordination	Vegetable Oils Cottonseed Corn Soybean, Nuts Legumes
Magnesium	Fatigue Insomnia Anxiety Hyperactivity Anger Tremors Numbness Tingling Rapid Pulse High Blood Pressure Heart Irregularities	Wheat Germ Almonds Cashews Brazil Nuts Soybeans Parsnips Oats Rye Corn
Calcium	High Blood Pressure Osteoporosis Muscle Pain Muscle Spasms Insomnia Nervousness Hyperactivity PMS	Milk Products Cheese Yogurt Canned Salmon Green Leafy Vegetables
Malic Acid	Muscle Pain Stiffness	Apples Fruits

Vitamin C is present in citrus fruits and functions as an antioxidant, it may have antibiotic-like qualities at higher doses, and assists the intestines in normal functioning. Vitamin B complex, present in green leafy vegetables, is essential for nerve transmission and healthy functioning of the nerves and liver. It affects sleep, mental capacity, heart and lung functions. Vitamin E, present in brown rice, kale, apricots, sunflower and pumpkin seeds, can improve circulation and cellular function. Magnesium, present in green leafy vegetables, legumes and nuts, is essential for muscle and heart functioning. It inhibits action of excitatory amino acids that lead to increased pain and discomfort. Magnesium levels are inversely related to pain/tenderness levels, the higher the magnesium levels in muscle cells, the lower the pain complaints. Calcium, present in milk products, is essential for muscle function as well as bone strength. Calcium-magnesium combination is an effective muscle relaxant and sleep inducer. Malic acid is a food acid present in apples and other fruits. It is important for cell function and energy production in cells. It can be obtained as magnesium malate. Vitamin B12, if deficient, can cause fatigue and anemia.

It is possible to swallow all the right nutrients but unless the stomach and intestines are able to digest the nutrients and allow optimal absorption into the bloodstream the nutrients cannot benefit the individual. The enteric nervous system directs the function of the stomach and intestines. With dysfunction of the enteric nervous system common in CPP there is often abnormal nutrient absorption. Self care and medications that normalize the enteric nervous system and gut function can lead to significantly less fatigue and pain. Foods and supplements that are more completely digested will make a difference in pain and fatigue as well. Fructose based vitamin and mineral supplements have been the most effective for some CPP individuals. Any supplement should break down in water within 20 minutes to be effectively digested in the gut. Some CPP individuals utilize nutrients better if food combining strategies are followed, such as eating protein and vegetables together or avoiding protein and starches in combination.

Exercise

Pelvic Muscle Force Field (PMFF) exercises are the foundation of an exercise program for CPP. The exercise series facilitates increased circulation to the region, improves resting levels and strength during contraction of the essential muscles. The PMFF core exercise develops coordinated synergistic sequencing of pelvic muscles in conjunction with obturator internus and adductors/internal rotators. Start with the Core Exercise and when it becomes easy and comfortable advance to PMFF exercises on page 193.

Core Exercise— Alternating Mid Range Hip External and Internal Rotation

The core exercise is alternating hip internal and external rotation in midrange. This exercise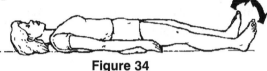

Figure 34

is performed in supine with knees bent or straight, in sitting, and standing. In standing, with toes pointed out, perform small range knee

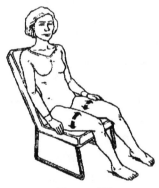

bends (1"-3"). In standing, with knees unlocked, rotate heels out (hip internal rotation) and in (hip external rotation). Perform this exercise in supine before getting out of bed in the morning and in the evening at bedtime. Perform the standing form of the core exercise while brushing your teeth and washing your face. The sitting form of the core exercise can be performed during work or while eating or watching TV.

Figure 35

When active exercise is easy and pain is decreased, resistance in the form of resistive balls and bands can be added. When resistance is added begin with 1-3 repetitions with resistance initially and gradually increase to 8-10 repetitions over a 7-14 day period.

Rolling the hips in and out lift the bladder and bowel into optimal position and maintain closure of the bladder outlet and bowel anorectal angle and sphincter. The pelvic floor muscles are synergistically activated without the individual consciously contracting them.

Medications

Medications are often recommended as part of the total management approach for CPP. See page 147 for a list of commonly used medications. Medications rarely eliminate all symptoms but often help with the sleep disorder and to decrease pain. To find the optimum medication combination, it may take the physician several trials of different medications in different amounts. Medication can be effective over an extended period. Medication may also lose its effectiveness after a period of time and need to be changed for another. Know what characteristics each medication has, its side effects, and how and when it should be taken. If there is more than one physician prescribing medication be sure that each physician knows all the medications being taken to avoid possible drug interactions. There are prescription guides available in bookstores or at the pharmacy to help you stay informed.

One last word about medication. Since CPP is a chronic condition, medications that help are frequently needed over an extended period of time and on a daily basis. There is a tendency for CPP individuals to take medication until they feel better and then quit taking it or take it infrequently. "I don't want to be dependent on drugs to feel good. I'm not someone who uses drugs," are commonly heard comments. The mind set that is needed when thinking about CPP and medications is that the individual has a lack of certain chemicals that then increase the fatigue and pain. The medications help replace those missing chemicals so the body can function optimally. They are often needed over the long term to help the CPP individual experience the fewest symptoms. Medication is one of the many tools an individual with CPP can use to help manage the symptoms of the illness and speed recovery. Stopping medications abruptly because of fears about drug use can cause a setback in treatment that is demoralizing. Medicine is not a crutch, it is an aid to ensuring improvement and should be respected as much as biofeedback or an exercise program. If an individual fears medication it is important to talk with the physician about the concerns.

Massage

Massage can be helpful for pain relief, improved circulation, relaxation of muscles and removal of waste product build up. Massage needs to start gently; pain is not gain in fibromyalgia. As the muscles release, deeper massage may be appropriate. Special techniques, including craniosacral and myofascial release techniques, can be appropriate and beneficial. Massage therapists, physical therapists, occupational therapists, nurses, and chiropractors are all individuals trained in massage.

Self massage or having a family member massage areas can be effective using essential oils and light to moderate stroking over muscle areas that are painful or tight. The touch helps quiet and relax the muscles and the essential oils help increase circulation, decrease pain and tightness. It is important to avoid trying to "dig out" the pain with deep, intense massage techniques which will often increase the symptoms. The pain does not have to get worse before it can get better.

To reach hard to get areas use two tennis balls in a sock and place the balls between the individual and the floor to massage a particular spot for 1-3 minutes to decrease pain. Two racket balls in a sock fit the low back better than tennis balls. There are various canes and knobs on the market to help you reach difficult spots. Hiring a professional massage therapist for a weekly massage is also beneficial. Interview them first, to make sure they understand the needs of chronic pelvic pain.

Acupressure / Acupuncture Therapy

Acupressure and acupuncture are non-medicinal ways to help control pain. Acupressure uses pressure rather than needles to treat key areas of the body. Acupressure can be performed by the individual or a friend by applying pressure with the middle finger or thumb to acupressure points. A physical therapist, massage therapist, chiropractor or physician may have the training for acupressure treatment.

Acupuncture is a form of Chinese medicine in which inserting fine needles into the skin of the ear, the feet or other body parts relieves chronic pain, fatigue or other neurological symptoms. Pain relieving brain chemicals called endorphins and enkephalins are released during acupuncture. These chemicals block the pain circuits from sending their message to the brain so "you don't feel the pain." Acupuncture has few side effects if disposable, standard needles are used and are administered by a trained acupuncturist. Pain relief should be felt within 5-10 treatments. Acupuncture can be used to improve the associated symptom related to FMS as well as the pain. Treating the Chinese organs or meridians of spleen, liver, kidney, lung and heart through acupuncture can be beneficial in relieving CPP symptoms. Physician acupuncturists and licensed acupuncturists are qualified to administer this treatment.

Tender Point Pressure

Direct pressure using the thumb or a finger for 7-8 seconds, is one beneficial technique. Direct pressure over acupressure sites for 7-8 seconds can be effective for pain relief and easy to do several times a day. (Figure 36)

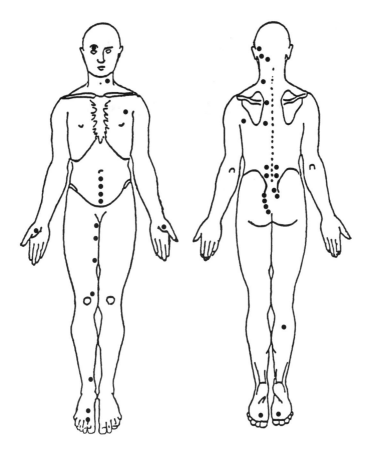

Figure 36: Acupressure Sites

Oils and Lotions

A number of lotions, creams and oils can be used in combination with medication to ease muscle pain and tightness. Especially for those individuals who are drug sensitive, oils and lotions don't cause stomach or gastrointestinal irritation or the side effects of some medications yet they can give relief from pain and muscle tightness.

Essential oil mixtures in a base oil such as almond oil can be easily applied to painful areas by the individual or family member. Specific oils decrease pain, detoxify waste products and improve circulation. Commonly used essential oils include lavender, lemon, rosemary, juniper, and bergamot.

Lotions containing capsaicin are known to decrease substance P. Capsaicin is derived from red peppers and produces a hot, burning sensation when rubbed into the skin. Repeated application to a specific area over a week can result in decreased pain. Capsaicin is not used over the labia, vulva, or scrotum area. Extra virgin olive oil is beneficial for vulvadynia/vulvar vestibulitis.Other lotions produce a cooling effect on the skin for relief of pain and discomfort.

Self Talk – Positive Self Statements

The mind is always saying something positive, negative, or neutral as an individual goes through the day. Even while sleeping at night there are thoughts and dreams. Self talk can be helpful or hurtful in relation to CPP symptoms and an individual's accomplishments. To develop an awareness of what self talk is like, for one or two days pause four or five times during the day and jot down what thoughts are present at that time in relation to what you are doing and how you are feeling. Are there primarily positive or negative thoughts? Are there repetitive thoughts? Now take the positive thoughts and repeat them throughout the day such as every time breathing practice is scheduled or every time you talk on the phone. Pair the positive self statement with some event that occurs frequently in the day. If there is negative self talk, substitute positive statements for the negative thoughts.

Examples of positive self statements are:

- I am healing, I am healing more each moment of each day.
- I am trying, I am doing the best I can.

- I deserve to be healthy and happy, I am healthy and happy.
- I feel quiet and calm, I am quiet and calm.
- I love you, I will take care of you.

For some individuals positive self statements seem like lies or half truths. If that occurs, put "I am trying" or "I am beginning to" in front of the statement. Remember every thought stimulates biochemical and electrical events in the brain and gut which then flow to every cell of the body and affect all other body and mind functions.

Rest is a Treatment Essential in CPP

Rest is a vital part of anyone's daily schedule, usually accomplished at an unconscious level. Relaxing into a chair for a few minutes between jobs, reading the newspaper or watching television and dozing off for a short period, sitting under a tree and gazing at the clouds during lunch time, or sitting at your desk stretching towards the ceiling while releasing two or three big sighs are all forms of rest the body and mind need and ask for throughout the day. Rest is necessary for energy conservation and a return to neutrality and slow idle before going on to a new task.

Both mind and body rest are important to accomplish during the slow idle periods throughout the day. Mind rest techniques can include meditation, positive self talk, and breathing awareness to name a few. Body rest includes skeletal muscle release and internal organ systems' quieting using Physiological Quieting techniques such as breathing and hand warming. The need for supportive, comfortable chairs, couches and beds that enable the individual's muscles to let go into a relaxed state with minimal pain are important for body rest.

Mind and body rest needs to occur frequently throughout the day for short periods. Sometimes it will only be a minute or so of breathing and quiet muscle release, other times 5 minutes of focused meditation, and at least 20-30 minutes of extended mind and body rest using Physiological Quieting techniques once a day. When setting up a schedule for the day, **rest periods are as important as work periods**. These rest periods help ensure that the CPP tendency for elevated resting levels of muscle activity, autonomic nervous system activity and mental activity are frequently returned to more normal levels, to a slow idle. These rest periods can be essential in maintaining a decreased pain and fatigue level throughout the day instead of the pattern of a small window of relief in the morning with escalating pain and fatigue levels for the remainder of the day.

Pacing – Energy Management

Pacing is the breaking up of the day into multiple work, rest, and play sections. To pace the day it is important to first make a list of the work related tasks for the day and prioritize the top three while putting the others off until tomorrow. Pacing is breaking each of those jobs or tasks into two or three parts with planned rest periods in between.

Pacing is never finishing one job before you start a part of another one. Instead it means performing the first part of job one, then resting, then going to the first part of job two, then resting, then completing the first part of job three, then resting, then going back to the second part of job one, etc. With this kind of pacing, different muscles and different body postures are used for each new job. Fatigue is less of a problem because parts of jobs are done with frequent changes in muscle action and postural alignment. Frequent short rest periods with conscious return to neutral mind and body activity enables the CPP individual to accomplish more tasks with less fatigue and pain.

Daily Job List

1. Sweep floors
2.
3.
4.
5.
6.
7.

Daily Priority Jobs

1. Sweep floors
   a. part one: Sweep 1/2 kitchen floor
   b. part two: Sweep 1/2 kitchen floor
   c. part three: Sweep laundry room
2.
   a. part one:
   b. part two:
   c. part three:
3.
   a. part one:
   b. part two:
   c. part three:

Rest Activities

- Listening to music while reclining.
- Reading in supported sitting.
- Physiological Quieting.
- Meditation

Initially the rest cycles may be longer than work cycles, but gradually the two will become equal and eventually the work cycle can exceed the rest cycle and still maintain the goals of decreased pain and fatigue. For example:

Rest Cycle	Work Cycle
10 minutes	3-5 minutes
	increase 1-2 minutes/week
10 minutes	10 minutes
10 minutes	15 minutes

Play and Fun

Pacing means placing play and laughter into the work-rest routine throughout the day, not just when all work has been accomplished. **Play and laughter are required treatments multiple times during each day.** With that being the case, short periods of play will be scheduled into mid morning, mid afternoon, and evening. On some occasions, segments can be as simple and short as reading the funnies in the paper every morning and making sure to practice belly laughing. There needs to be a daily 20-30 minute play period with friends over tea, or spending 20 minutes in a hot bath or hot tub, going to the movie, or watching a favorite TV program.

Some individuals, when asked what they do for fun, respond "work." It is necessary to begin making a master list of play and fun activities that are not work related so you can vary the play activities on a daily and weekly basis and continue to be on the lookout for a new play or fun activity to add to the list. Try to find a new one every week or two. Watch other people and catch them having fun, see what they are doing. It means that play and laughter have equal weight with work and rest in a daily schedule.

Pacing of work, rest and play can be easily monitored by using a daily journal. As part of a nightly routine fill in the day's activities and summarize where pacing went well. (Figure 37)

DAILY JOURNAL OF PLAY, REST, WORK

Date_____

Time	Play	Rest	Work
A.M. 7:00-8:00 8:00-9:00 9:00-10:00			(ea. task = 3 parts) (3-4 tasks/day)

Figure 37

Play Activity List

- Tea with friends
- Favorite video
- Reading the funnies
- _____

- _____
- _____
- _____
- _____

Prioritizing

Prioritizing is making decisions – decisions that some work is more important to do today, that some work is more important to do next week and some work you should never do but rather give to someone else or let it go undone. Prioritizing is listing all the work titles you have and the roles you carry out under each of those, then making decisions as to which are important to be done on a daily, weekly, monthly or never ever basis. It needs to be emphasized that prioritizing is done in the context of the pacing schedule you have already planned. **Prioritizing is more important than getting all your work roles accomplished. Figure out how the work roles can fit into your optimum pacing schedule.**

Work Titles I Fulfill	**Roles**
	Examples:
■ Parent to children	■ Transporter
■ Parent to elderly parents	■ House cleaner
(list specifics)	
■ Spouse	■ Listener/emotional support
■ Banker, teacher, teller etc.	■ Money transfer, reaching, grasp
■ Volunteer	
■ Friend	

Pain Relieving Modalities

Pain relief is the number one priority for most individuals with chronic pelvic pain. Effective techniques may be different for each person. Examples of pain relieving modalities include:

Heat

The benefits from 20-30 minutes of heat include increased circulation and decreased muscle tightness. Moist heat pads are usually preferred over dry heating pads. The moist heating pad purchased at the drug store will often have little sponges that are moistened. Medical supply stores have heating pads that draw moisture from the air. They are a little more costly but are larger and conform better to the body contours. A damp towel or commercial hot pack heated in the microwave or in hot water for a few minutes is another good way to get moist heat. Hot water in the form of a hot tub, hot shower, or whirlpool bath is always a good choice. Hot tubs need to be under 102° F to allow an individual to stay in the water comfortably and safely for 20-30 minutes.

Cold

Some individuals benefit from ice so it is worth a try even if it sounds uncomfortable. One form of treatment is an ice massage to a painful area. Freeze water in an 8 oz. paper cup, then tear away the top edge of paper so the ice can be moved around the palm size painful area for about five minutes. Initially it feels very cold but within five minutes the area will be numb. Use a towel to catch the drips. Some

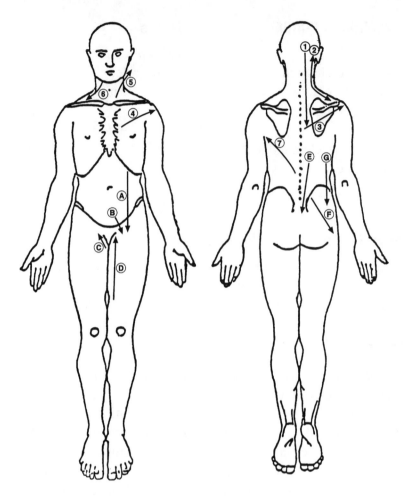

Figure 38: Vapocoolant Spray Techniques

individuals find it more tolerable to use ice while in a hot tub or shower or while they have heat on another part of the body. If cold hands are a problem, use gloves and a styrofoam cup.

An ice pack is another form of cold application. Commercial ice packs and ice probes are available through medical supply stores. Ice packs can be homemade using a wet or dry towel wrapped around a package of frozen peas or corn or crushed ice. A frozen wet towel provides more intense cold. A ten minute application of an ice pack is usually adequate.

Cold Spray – Heat

This technique is designed to obtain effective pain relief and increased motion in affected body areas. Vapocoolant spray is a cold, fine spray of gas under pressure. It is prescribed by a physician for clinic and/or home use. At home it is initially used for 7-10 days to decrease symptoms and then it is used as needed during acute exacerbations or after exercise. For use with CPP, body segments are treated instead of one or two specific muscles and the body position during the treatment is more midline than stretched as it is when myofascial muscle shortening is being treated. The term "midline spray and heat" is used rather than the more common term "spray and stretch." Initially a physician or therapist can use the technique as part of the office visit to evaluate effectiveness and improve pain and limited range of motion. If the technique is effective, the health care professional can demonstrate the techniques to a support person so a home program can be done 1-2 times daily during painful flare-ups (Figure 38). When pain is primarily in the lower body, (low back, hips, buttocks, legs, abdomen) the spray techniques A-G are completed bilaterally.

Alternate – Heat – Ice

Some individuals get the most benefit from using a combination of heat and ice. Use heat (heating pad, hot tub) for 7-10 minutes, then cold (ice pack, ice probe) for 3-5 minutes, and then heat for 7-10 minutes.

Heat – Stretch and Ice – Heat

This technique is designed to obtain an effective stretch of a tight muscle group without setting off muscle spasms. Heat the muscle group for about three minutes, then put that area on a gentle stretch and hold the stretch while rubbing an ice cup or ice edge in lines about 1/2 inch apart parallel to the muscle fibers under the skin. Keep the stretch gentle and steady for 30-60 seconds then heat the area again for approximately three minutes.

Journaling

The habit of regularly writing in a blank book or on pages in a notebook can be helpful in tracking the ups and downs of CPP, in seeing small steps of progress that lead to improved health, and in relieving the "free floating" anxiety CPP individuals describe.

Journaling is "stream of conscious" writing. There is no right or wrong way to do it. Just open the blank book or take some note paper and write whatever flows from the mind and hand. No one needs to read it or judge it. Let the mind empty all its thoughts, worries, and concerns on the paper. When the censor part of the mind tries to stop the thought flow to the paper, remember this writing is not for judging, it is for releasing feeling and thoughts.

In CPP at times the brain activity for thoughts, worries, and ideas becomes excessive, getting in the way of everyday life just as the muscles become overactive causing pain and fatigue. The overactive brain leads to feelings of anxiety, confusion, indecision, and mental paralysis. Releasing any and all thoughts to paper assists in quieting brain activity.

Journaling can be done day or night. Keep notebooks on a bed stand and in a purse. Some CPP individuals are not able to write so a computer or audio or video tape recorder is a better mode of communication.

A second type of daily journal is designed to give a picture of patterns and relationships between symptoms, work, exercise, rest, and sleep. On a longitudinal 24 hour scale the CPP individual keeps track of pain levels, sleep hours, number of awakenings at night, work, rest, and exercise cycles. See the Weekly Self Care Report (Figure 21). Progress or problems can be seen more easily with this type of journaling.

It can be helpful to keep a daily journal to pick up patterns and relationships between symptoms and daily activities and stressors. In the journal the CPP individual keeps track of pain, stiffness and fatigue levels during morning, noon, afternoon and evening, medication taken, menstrual cycle pattern, exercise level, and jobs done.

The goal for CPP individuals is to modify activities or stressors that increase symptoms so there is an equilibrium achieved for extended periods of time. The equilibrium is often not a completely pain-free state, nor totally fatigue-free, but interventions throughout the day keep the equilibrium. A self care routine with regular mini reassessments of mind-body function are essential to attain that steady state of equilibrium.

Crisis Management Program

Flare-ups or exacerbations are going to occur in CPP even with the best management program. A prearranged crisis management plan will help the CPP individual deal with the flare-ups. The crisis management plan is comprised of items that have worked in the past in order of priority, a list of support people to contact, and positive self statements that direct the mind and body towards health and healing.

Examples of Crisis Management Plan

Alter the day's plans to fit your needs!

- Use modalities such as hot shower or hot tub for 20 minutes.
- Take 20 minutes 2-3 times today for Physiological Quieting.
- Use pain relieving oil or lotion on affected muscles.
- . Do breathing and hand warming every half hour to hour.
- Take a relaxing walk with a friend.
- Take medication as directed for crisis times.
- Increase rest cycle length in the daily plan.
- Emphasize positive self statements.
- Evaluate life stressors, i.e., environmental, emotional.
- Consult with therapist or physician if not improved in 48 hours.

My Crisis Management Plan

1. _____

2. _____

3. _____

4. _____

5. _____

Chapter 16

Advanced Techniques

Once the General Self Care Stabilizing Loop has been successfully integrated into daily life additional, more advanced techniques can be of benefit to the individual with CPP. The Advanced Self Care Techniques are designed to continue the progression towards independence and integration into daily activities without pain as a limitation. Begin slowly, using one advanced technique at a time. After several days to a week using the new technique assess its benefits for the short and long term life goals. Continue to add other advanced techniques making sure each is integrated into life as a positive self care behavior. Record and monitor the advanced techniques on the Master Tests and Self-Care Stabilizing Record. (Figure 39)

Advanced Self Care Techniques

Physiological Quieting
    Body-Mind Synchrony
    Pelvic Warming
Positive Self Statements
Pelvic Muscle Force Field
   Exercises
Postural Exercises
Stretching Techniques
Therapeutic Ball Exercises
Pool Exercises
Hip Elevation

Dietary/Environmental Irritants
Nutrition
Bowel Program
Acupressure/Massage
Foot Massage/Exercise
Healing Oils/Creams
Modalities
Myofascial Release
Visceral Mobility
PTSD Techniques

My Master Test and Self Care Stabilizing Record														
Tests: Date														
1.														
2.														
3.														
4.														
Self Care Protocol														
1.														
2.														
3.														
4.														
5.														
6.														
7.														
8.														
9.														
10.														

Figure 39

Advanced Physiological Quieting (APQ)

Physiological Quieting normalizes the messages from the body to the brain, the brain to the body, and between different organs and tissues. The basic PQ techniques include hand warming, diaphragmatic breathing, and body-mind quieting designed to open the communication loop between the body and the brain. The advanced PQ techniques include body-brain energy synchrony and pelvic warming. These techniques are designed to synchronize the brain and body electrical activity. Fehmi describes synchrony of brain wave patterns as open focus®. In contrast to left-brain hemisphere narrow focus processing, open focus brain wave synchrony is a diffuse focus, an effortless awareness by the right brain hemisphere. Left hemisphere narrow focus is comparable to memorizing a list of anatomy terms. Right hemisphere open focus is comparable to a lion reclined on a hill, alert and relaxed and watching the plains below. This attention difference is reflected in brain wave changes. Narrow focus attention is 20 hertz, beta brain waves. Open focus® attention is 8-12 hertz, alpha brain waves and theta brain waves 4-8 hertz. Open focus® attention techniques are designed to broaden the brain's attention to peripheral awareness and to bring synchrony of energy in all parts of the brain. Advanced Physiological Quieting takes open focus® concepts one step further. Advanced Physiological Quieting is designed to bring synchrony of energy patterns to body centers in conjunction with brain centers. This is accomplished through focus on body systems and mind imagining. Fehmi's research describes the concept of "imagining space" as producing alpha waves in the brain. Advanced Physiological Quieting is designed to integrate the synchrony of those brain waves with body system energy cycles. For example, the heart energy system and the gut energy system become synchronized with the head brain energy system. This allows efficient communication between the body and brain for optimal health.

To practice APQ Body-Brain Synchrony:
- Imagine the space around your pelvis.
- Imagine the space within your pelvis.
- Imagine the space to the right of your pelvis, to the left of your pelvis.
- Imagine the space on top of your pelvis, below your pelvis.
- Imagine the space in front of your pelvis, in back of your pelvis.
- Imagine clouds of space within your pelvis.

Repeat this sequence using the organs of heart, lungs, uterus, ovaries, bladder, bowel, intestines, and stomach. Repeat this sequence using the skeletal structures of sacrum, low back, and hips. Repeat this sequence using the soft tissue structures of pelvic muscles, buttocks muscles, back muscles, and hip muscles.

Pelvic Warming

Pelvic warming is another APQ technique. When handwarming becomes easy, progress to pelvic warming. Pelvic warming is an effective way to decrease CPP pain when ischemia is a factor. Even a slight increase in internal pelvic temperature can be related to a decrease in pelvic pain and muscle relaxation.

To practice APQ Pelvic Warming:

- Use a surface thermister placed in the leg crease area of the groin. Monitor the temperature at the beginning and end of this exercise.

- Focus attention in the lower pelvis.

- Think to yourself: "My pelvic area is warmer and warmer. Warmth is flowing into my pelvic area, warmer and warmer."

- Visualize in your mind's eye the warmest color surrounding the pelvic area, penetrating deep into the pelvis. Feel the warmth of that color warming the area, warmer and warmer.

- Imagine yourself in the warmest, safest place. Feel the warmth of that place flow into your pelvic area, warmer and warmer.

- Think to yourself: "My pelvic area is warmer and warmer."

Advanced Positive Self Statements
Talking to Yourself

An individual talks to him/herself with an internal dialogue on a regular basis. What an individual says will determine to some extent the quality and direction of life according to Butler. The mind is always saying something positive, negative, or neutral throughout the day. Even while sleeping there are thoughts and dreams. This internal dialogue influences every cell of the body, every organ function, and all pain and comfort levels.

Butler describes that when self talk is analyzed the thoughts can be divided into three judging categories: commands (drivers), prohibitions (stoppers), and faulty thinking (confusers). The drivers include: "be perfect," "hurry up," "be strong," "please others," "try hard." These drivers refuse to allow an individual freedom to listen to internal needs and respond to them. These internal needs could include: "I'm tired, I need a nap." "I want to try something new and learn by doing and making mistakes." "I want to begin this activity but not necessarily finish it today." When permitters are substituted for drivers in internal dialogue, freedom and health can return to the body and mind.

Stoppers include: catastrophizing, negative self labeling, setting rigid requirements, and don't statements. These stoppers refuse to allow an individual freedom to create new visions of the self, explore the interaction of others' thoughts and ideas with their own, or experiment with being "different." When permitters and the words "even if" are substituted for stoppers in self talk, freedom and health can return to the body and mind.

Confusers include: arbitrary inferences, misattribution, cognitive deficiency, over generalization, either/or thinking, vague language, and magnification. When actions are based on arbitrary, not fact based, evidence, internal dialogue can be negative, hurtful and simply not truthful. When either/or thinking forces one into a box of being either perfect or no good the impossibility of life creates stress that increases pain and organic dysfunction. Misattribution implies that someone else is to blame or is responsible for the individual's feelings rather than the individual being responsible for his/her own reaction to an event. Cognitive deficiency implies a narrow perception of a complex situation. "I did not get the job because I wasn't cute." Magnification means amplifying the importance of an event or situation. A young woman loses her glasses in the lake and sobs uncontrollably for hours. When "I" messages state feelings and opinions, confusers are eliminated. "Bringing it down to size" and the technique of using the prefix of "right now, I feel" can eliminate confusers, according to Butler.

The language of self support includes I messages, self affirmations, buffers, and permissions.

"I love you, I will take care of you," is an I message and an affirmation.

"I deserve to sleep when I am tired," is an I message and a permission.

"I am learning with each small step I take. I am not a failure." is a buffer.

The first step in developing positive self talk is taking an inventory of the internal dialogue that occurs on a daily basis (Figure 40). Write down what goes through the mind. Then group these thoughts into positive and negative categories. For every negative thought determine if it is a driver, a stopper or a confuser. Then write a positive antidote for each negative thought. Now take the positive thoughts and repeat them throughout the day. Pair them with other activities such as every time teeth are brushed or the phone is answered.

Examples of positive self statements include:
"I am healing, I am healing more each moment of each day."
"I am trying, I am doing the best I can."
"I deserve to be health and happy. I am healthy and happy."
"I deserve to sleep through the night. I sleep through the night and feel rested."

For some individuals positive self statements seem like lies or half truths. If that occurs, put "I am trying" or "I am beginning to" in front of the statement. Remember every thought stimulates biochemical and electrical events in the brain and gut which then flow to every cell of the body and affect all other body and mind functions.

Build a pyramid of self statements. Begin with statements already present in the mind and gradually develop more positive and futuristic self talk.

Inventory of Self Talk

1._____

2._____

3._____

4._____

5._____

6._____

Positive Self Talk   Negative Self Talk

1._____   1._____

2._____   2._____

3._____   3._____

Pyramid of Positive Self Talk

_____

_____

_____

_____

Figure 40 Self Talk Pyramid

Advanced Pelvic Muscle Force Field Exercises

Level 1 – Breathing diaphragm and transverse abdominus action
Level 2 – Lower leg and foot muscle action
Level 3 – Head, neck and shoulder muscle action
Level 4 – Whole body facilitation
Level 5 – Standing rotation facilitation

Once the core PMFF exercises are easy the advanced PMFF exercises can be initiated. These advanced exercises integrate the breathing diaphragm, transverse abdominus, lower leg and foot musculature, shoulder and forearm musculature with the PMFF. These advanced exercises integrate cranial movements and craniosacral rhythm with PMFF function. There are five levels of Advanced PMFF Exercises for CPP.

Advanced PMFF Exercise – Level 1

Breathing Diaphragm and Transverse Abdominus Action

Level 1 – Advanced PMFF Exercise includes integrating the breathing diaphragm and abdominal muscles with action of the

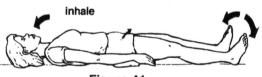

inhale

Figure 41

PMFF. Inhale as the hips externally rotate and relax the abdominal muscles. Exhale through pursed lips as the hips internally rotate. (Figure 41 & 42)

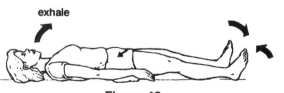

exhale

Figure 42

During inhale the breathing diaphragm descends into the abdominal region, the a b d o m i n a l musculature relaxes, and the abdominal contents expand into the relaxed space. During exhale, the breathing diaphragm ascends, synergistically facilitating contraction of the transverse abdominus. The transverse abdominus and PMFF synergistically contract.

Advanced PMFF Exercise – Level 2

Lower Leg and Foot Muscle Action

Level 2 – Advanced PMFF Exercise integrates the lower leg and foot muscles with action of the PMFF. As the hips roll out with inhale, dorsiflex the ankles and abduct and extend the toes. As the hips roll in with exhale, plantarflex the ankles and adduct and flex the toes.

The chain of interconnected fasciae extend from the PMFF to the toes. The obturator internus and its fascia share fibers with the sacrotuberous and sacrospinous ligaments which share fibers with the biceps femoris which attaches to the head of the fibula and is associated with the fascial and ligamentous connections of the distal tibiofibular joint, navicular and fifth metatarsal. Foot and ankle movements through this fascial bridge affect the length-tension relationship of the PMFF and thus bladder and bowel position and function.

The distal nerves of the lumbosacral plexus (2, 3, 4) innervate the intrinsic muscles of the toes and also innervate the PMFF and the bowel and bladder. Fanning or abducting and adducting the toes facilitates PMFF action through interneuron connections at the spinal cord level and through retrograde stimulation of the common nerve roots.

Advanced PMFF Exercise- Level 3

Head, Neck and Shoulder Muscles

Level 3 – Advanced PMFF Exercise includes integrating the head, neck and shoulder muscles with action of the PMFF. Tip the chin up several degrees and roll the shoulders out during hip outward rotation. Drop the chin and roll the shoulders in during hip inward rotation. The head rocks on the upper cervical vertebrae in a small, slow motion. When the elbows are straight, thumbs roll up with hip outward rotation and roll down with hip inward rotation. Incorporate these motions with Levels 1 and 2 actions of breathing, abdominal and leg and foot motions.

The nerve roots of the parasympathetic division of the ANS exit from cranial and sacral locations. Facilitating optimal function of this division encourages more normal PMFF and bladder and bowel resting tone. It assists in the balance of sympathetic and parasympathetic action affecting body functions.

Shoulder girdle motion and shoulder rotation facilitate synergistic action of the PMFF through their fascial connections. Shoulder girdle fascia interconnects with the fascia of ribs and breathing diaphragm which integrates with abdominal and visceral fascia as well as the endopelvic fascia of the PMFF.

Advanced PMFF Exercise – Level 4

Whole Body Facilitation of PMFF

Level 4 - Whole Body Facilitation of PMFF incorporates the core exercise with levels 1-3 muscle activities.
- Inhale – External Rotation of Shoulders and Hips
- Head Extension (O/A)
- Foot Dorsiflexion, Toe Abduction and Extension
- Exhale – Internal Rotation of Shoulders and Hips
- Head Flexion (O/A)
- Foot Plantar Flexion, Toe Adduction and Flexion

Posture

Standing and sitting posture is the base from which most movement occurs in adults. In CPP during standing it is common to see forward head, elevated, rounded shoulders, knees extended and weight acceptance on one leg more than another. The shoulder and neck muscles are over-active and seem to hold the body up. The head and shoulders often lead during walking.

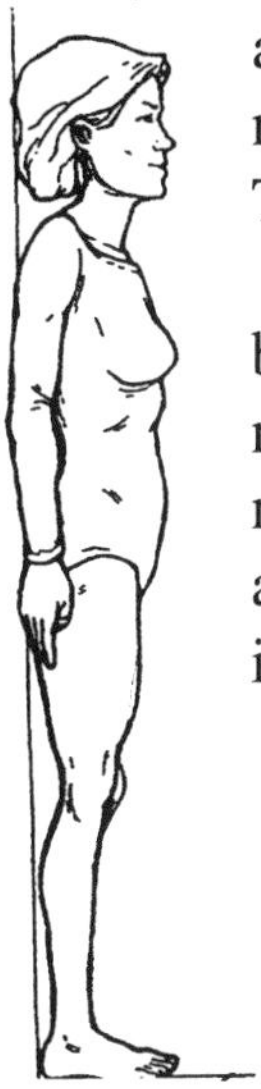

It is important to understand that standing posture should be maintained primarily by the bony skeleton and ligaments, not muscle action. There is minimal activity of the ankle muscles to maintain balance; the shoulder muscles, the abdominal and buttocks muscles should be relaxed. To stand in the most effective pain-free posture:
- Take weight equally on both feet.
- Unlock both knees.
- Push the top back of the head towards the clouds. Let the chin drop slightly as the spine lengthens.
- Release shoulders, thinking of the shoulder and neck muscles as a velvet cloak resting on a hanger (the

Figure 43

skeleton).
- Release jaw, teeth apart, tongue released from the roof of the mouth.
- Slow, low diaphragmatic breath in the low abdomen. (Figure 43)

Once the standing posture is comfortable, progress to:
- Weight shift in small amplitudes side to side.
- Perform slow, small knee bends.
- Weight shift front to back with one foot in front of the other.

During these exercises, lead with the hips, keeping the shoulders and neck released and relaxed. Maintain slow, low diaphragmatic breathing.

Advanced PMFF Exercise – Level 5

Standing Rotation Facilitation of PMFF

Level 5 - When standing posture and the core PMFF exercises are easily accomplished this exercise can be done to improve sacro-iliac stability, balance, and gait.
- Stand with feet apart and toes pointed out a few degrees.
- Unlock the knees and maintain them in slight flexion throughout the exercise.
- Bring both hands to the right hip with exhale, then back to center with inhale.
- Bring both hands to the left hip with exhale, then back to center with inhale.

This rotates the trunk on the pelvis and activates the transverse abdominus and PMFF.

- Rotate the right foot on the heel.
- Rotate the right foot out with inhale and in with exhale.
- Rotate the left foot out with inhale and in with exhale.

This rotates the lower extremity on the pelvis and activates the PMFF.

Combine the two exercises into one. (Figure 44)
- Bring both hands to the right hip while rotating the right foot in with exhale.
- Bring both hands to the left hip while rotating the right foot out

with inhale.
- Return to midline.
- Bring both hands to the left hip while rotating the left foot in with exhale.
- Bring both hands to the right hip while rotating the left foot out with inhale.
- Return to midline.

This exercise facilitates action of the breathing diaphragm, transverse abdominus and PMFF in standing balance and gait pattern. It facilitates lumbar and sacroiliac stabilization during balance and gait.

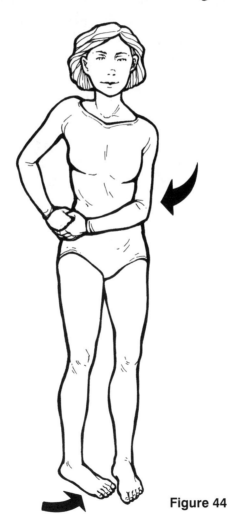

Figure 44

197

Stretching

The goal of stretching is to increase the ease of pain-free movement. For the individual with CPP the technique for stretching a tight muscle is different than a "feel good" full motion stretch. Stretching needs to be done when the body is warm and relaxed. This can be accomplished in a hot shower, after a warm bath, after 5-10 minutes of heat application, or following active exercise. Muscles need to be stretched slowly just until the beginning of discomfort is noted, concentrating on avoiding pain. Breathe into the stretch for 15-30 seconds. Think slow, small, soft, smooth, sensitive stretch. The breath is low, use diaphragmatic breathing. Stretching to "pull out" the tightness doesn't work. It can set off more muscle tightening. Return to neutral slowly and smoothly to avoid rebound tightening. One to three repetitions is enough. The typical stretch to the end of range with overpressure sets off the already overactive stretch reflex and feeds into the high resting tone (gamma bias) present in CPP muscles. Figure 45 shows appropriate shower stretches.

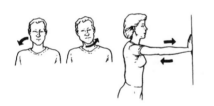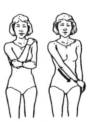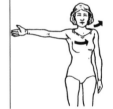

Figure 45: Shower Stretches

The goals of stretching can be accomplished through positional stretches. Positional stretches are each held for 3-5 minutes while resting on a mat or bed. (Figure 46)

A few stretches or exercises at lunch and coffee breaks help relax the muscles that have been used during work and increase blood flow to the area while decreasing tension. Another good time for the individual to take a few minutes for him/herself is after work and before tackling the evening activities. Taking 15-20 minutes between work and dinner to recline using positional stretches can help. When not working outside the home, it is important to develop a daily routine. In addition to bed and shower stretches, doing some stretches and exercises after breakfast, mid morning, after lunch and before dinner helps with pain and stiffness. Another approach is to set a timer and do exercises every two hours for 3-5 minutes.

Midline Stretch

This technique is effective for CPP that is characterized by tender points and/or is suspected to be visceral referred pain and/or muscle spasm. Use heat for 1-3 minutes in the area of symptoms, for example the lower abdomen or groin. A thermophore is an effective and light weight form of heat. Focus on slow, diaphragmatic breathing. With inhale, rotate the hips or trunk slowly and smoothly just 3°-5° to one side. Rest in that position for 2 to 3 slow, low breaths releasing any muscle tightness with each exhale. Return slowly to the midline position with the next breath. Rest for a slow breath. Repeat three times to one side, then three times to the other side. Then assess the pain-free-range available that previously was limited by the tender point musculature. This "midline stretch" resets the gamma bias of the muscle spindle resulting in improved range of motion and decreased pain.

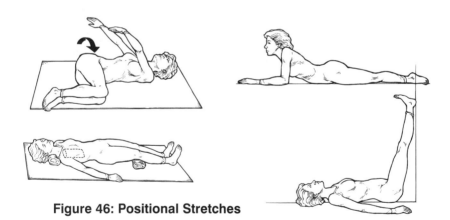

Figure 46: Positional Stretches

Therapeutic Ball Exercises

Therapeutic ball exercises are often beneficial for CPP due to sensory and proprioceptive feedback that the ball and gentle movement provide to the central and peripheral nervous system. Equilibrium reactions in conjunction with joint approximation and reflex inhibition of pelvic muscles can significantly improve pelvic and low back muscle function while facilitating normal breathing patterns and improving circulation.

Therapeutic ball exercises include (Figure 47)**:**

- Sitting: weight shifts front to back and side to side.
- Sitting: bounce gently into the ball..
- Prone: shift front to back and side to side.
- Sitting: roll knees out with inhale and in with exhale.

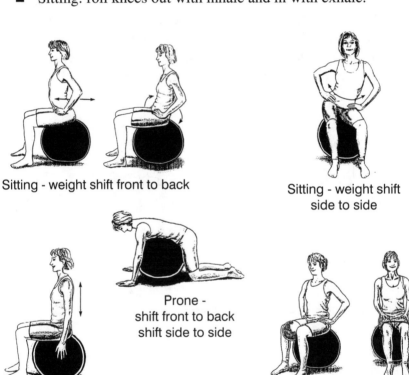

Sitting - weight shift front to back

Sitting - weight shift side to side

Prone - shift front to back shift side to side

Sitting - bounce gently

Sitting - roll knees inward roll knees outward

Figure 47: Therapeutic Ball Exercises

Pool Exercises

Most exercises can be accomplished with less pain and faster progression if done in a warm pool. Aerobic exercise is also very effective in shoulder level warm water. The recommended target heart rate is approximately 20% less than recommended target heart rate for aerobic exercise on land. Aerobic endurance improves from 3-5 minutes for the acutely painful CPP individual to 45 minutes with 1-2 rest periods when the pain and fatigue has decreased. There should be no pain during pool exercise. The CPP individual should feel better at the end of the session even though there is a tired feeling. It is common for an individual to comment that it seems so easy in the pool. It is important not to overdo initially. Build up gradually. Always keep warm, using a hot tub or sauna and warm shower before and after the exercises. The pool temperature is best between 87°-92° F to increase circulation and improve muscle relaxation. Being shoulder height in water eliminates 80% of gravity's pull on the body so movement can be the most efficient and pain-free. The water pressure decreases from the bottom up so there is a natural upward pressure that improves circulation in lower extremities to the heart.

Warm Up Stretches

(Don't forget to breathe.)
- Neck – forward/back to neutral, side bend, rotation
- Shoulders – hand to opposite shoulder
- Wrist – forward/back, circles each direction, turn palms up/down
- Leg/hip – hamstring stretch, Achilles stretch, roll knees out and in

Exercises in Standing

- Standing arm exercises while marching
  - Arms forward/backward
  - Hand circles
  - Hands to opposite shoulders
  - Arms forward & back - hand to face height
  - One hand on abdomen, one hand on low back, then reverse

- Elbows to shoulder height, then down
- Bend elbows, push down
■ Standing leg exercises
  - Marching
  - Weight shift side to side, feet apart
  - Rock forward (elbows back), rock back (arms forward)
  - Leg out to side
  - Leg back & forward
  - Leg circles

■ Arm and leg exercises
  - Hand to opposite knee
  - Hand toward opposite foot
  - Hand to inside heel
  - Hand to outside heel
  - Hands to right, legs to left – twist, then reverse

■ Water walking - forward, backward, side crossovers

Hip Elevation

If pelvic congestion or neurally mediated hypotension are factors in CPP, hip elevation can assist in draining the pelvic region of blood and lymph and decreasing pain. If pelvic organ descent, uterine prolapse, cystocele or rectocele, are factors in CPP, hip elevation can assist in repositioning the organs and other soft tissue and decreasing pain.

Once or twice a day elevate the hips higher than the heart using a foam wedge. (Figure 48) Remain in this position for approximately 15 minutes. During that time practice diaphragmatic breathing. Practice ankle pumps and core PMFF exercises.

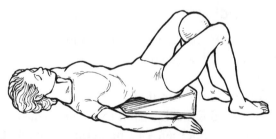

Figure 48: Hip Elevation

Any time pelvic pain begins to increase, recline and elevate the hips for 15 minutes, following the above procedures.

At night, sleep with the foot of the bed elevated 4-6 inches.

Dietary/Environmental Irritants and Substitutes

If CPP symptoms are related to dietary factors, strict elimination of these irritants should bring significant relief in 10-14 days. To reinforce the causative factor, reintroduce the eliminated food(s) and the CPP symptoms should return. Eliminate one food at a time. Always drink 6-8 glasses of water daily.

Dietary Irritants to the Bladder

Possible Irritants:

Alcoholic beverages	Citrus fruits	Cranberries	Tea
Apples	Coffee	Grapes	Tomatoes
Apple juice	Strawberries	Guava	Chocolate
Cantaloupe	Vinegar	Peaches	Vitamin B

Substitutions:

Low acid fruits	pears, apricots, papaya, watermelon
Coffee	Kava, cold brew from Starbucks, Pero
Tea	Non-citrus herbal, sun brewed tea
Vitamin C	Calcium carbonate co-buffered with calcium ascorbate

Dietary Irritants to the Bowel

	Substitute
Milk products	soy milk
Wheat products	rice flour, oat flour
Spicy foods	

Environmental Agents

Agent	**Substitute**
Hand and body soap	mild soaps without fragrance Neutrogena or Basis
Shampoo and cream rinses	wash hair in the sink so water does not run toward genitals

Detergents	no fabric rinses, no bleaches, mild soap
Douches	do not use
Feminine hygiene products	no vaginal deodorants, no scented tampons or sanitary pads
Clothing	avoid synthetic underwear, wear white, cotton underwear wash in Woolite and double rinse
Contraception	avoid condoms and contraceptive jellies, foams and creams
Newsprint	wash hands after reading newspaper
Medication	all drugs can cause allergic reaction so avoid or test
Toileting	wash hands before toilet time, use white toilet tissue, rinse Vulva with water after urinating

Nutrition

General nutrition guidelines for CPP and LBP were discussed in chapter fifteen. More specific suggestions for individual subcategory diagnoses are described here. Effective intervention for hypoglycemia, hypothyroid, and neurally mediated hypotension tendencies includes nutritional management. Nutritional changes should be discussed with the physician.

General Hypoglycemic Tendencies

Symptoms of General Hypoglycemia decrease with the elimination of simple sugars in the diet and an increase in complex carbohydrate consumption. Whole grains and vegetables are recommended instead of candy bars and colas even though cravings for these foods may be present. Consumption of fruit juice and white flour is not recommended.

Whole fruits like apples can be consumed in moderation – 1-2 a day. Avocados tend to depress insulin production so hypoglycemic tendencies can be improved with the consumption of avocados. Reducing meat protein while increasing complex carbohydrates is beneficial. Consuming complex carbohydrates every 3 hours can provide a more stable blood glucose level so 6 small meals a day, or 3 meals and 3 snacks is a better plan than 3 meals a day spaced 4-5 hours apart. It is important that individuals with hypoglycemic tendencies eat a small carbohydrate meal before going to bed at night. This helps to maintain the blood glucose levels through the night.

Vitamins and minerals can be helpful in hypoglycemia regulation. Chromium picolinate 300-600 mcg, vitamin B complex 50-100 mg, and coenzyme Q can all assist in stabilizing blood sugar levels. Zinc, 50 mg daily, is needed for insulin release from the pancreas. Herbs that may help hypoglycemic tendencies include bilberry and wild yam.

Self Care for General Hypoglycemia Tendencies

- Blood glucose testing multiple times/day
- Nutritional changes:
  - small meals every 2-3 hours
  - increase complex carbohydrates
  - refined sugars, fruit juice, white flour eliminated
  - vitamin/mineral boosters
    - chromium picolinate 300-600mcg
    - vitamin B complex 50-100mg
    - coenzyme Q 25-50mg
    - zinc 50mg
  - herb booster
    - bilberry
    - wild yam

Reactive Hypoglycemic Tendencies

Symptoms of Reactive Hypoglycemic Tendencies decrease with the elimination of simple sugars in the diet and an increase in fat and protein. Protein and fat intake slows the release of insulin in Reactive Hypoglycemia. Proteins break down into amino acids in the gut. It takes a much longer time to break down protein to amino acids than it takes to break down carbohydrates to glucose/sugar molecules. Amino acids stimulate different enteric nervous system responses than carbohydrates and glucose. Therefore, eating a relatively high protein breakfast could prevent the reactive hypoglycemic symptoms of fatigue, confusion, agitation, and pain. Instead the individual feels energized for the rest of the day.

Fat, similar to protein, slows the release of insulin. Fats break down into fatty acids in the gut. It takes longer to break down fat into fatty acids than it does to break down carbohydrates to glucose/sugar. Fatty acids stimulate different enteric nervous system responses than carbohydrates and glucose do. Therefore eating a relatively high fat diet can prevent the reactive hypoglycemic symptoms of fatigue, confusion, agitation, and pain.

Both protein and fat tend to set the enteric brake "on" so the pancreas is stimulated to release insulin and the small intestine is stimulated to release nutrients into the blood stream in a more graded, gradual fashion.

Combining carbohydrate, protein, and fat in each meal in a 40%, 30%, 30% ratio provides the enteric nervous system of the gut with the needed balance for more normal insulin release throughout the day. There is a need to eat frequently, usually every 2 hours. The first meal of the day sets the mood for the rest of the day. Just as Mary felt better when he ate a breakfast of eggs and bacon most individuals with Reactive Hypoglycemic Tendencies are better regulated the rest of the day if they have fat and protein for breakfast. Still others with Reactive Hypoglycemic Tendencies do better if there is an emphasis on fat with a serving of fruit to start the day. For example, a smoothie made of cream and fruit with no added sugar can set the enteric brake "on" at the beginning of the day and influence the rest of the day compared to eating cereal for breakfast which can set the enteric brake "off" and influence the rest of the day detrimentally. It is important to eat soon after getting up so blood glucose doesn't drop while you are getting ready for the day. A bedtime snack containing some fat slows the absorption levels of glucose into the blood stream during the night which helps maintain adequate glucose levels throughout the sleeping time. The Zone Diet books may be helpful resources for menus and dietary suggestions.

The same vitamins, minerals and herbs can be helpful in reactive hypoglycemia regulation as are helpful in general hypoglycemia.

Specific suggestions given by patients include:

- Yams and asparagus are good to eat when I am having problems with my intestines shutting down. They seem to respond within 24 hours in a comfortable way not an explosive over response that I would get with other foods or medications I tried.
- Smoothies made of fruit and cream have helped me get the day started on the right foot. I have a blueberry/ strawberry/ raspberry with cream smoothie in the morning, about 6-8 ounces for breakfast and then 3-4 ounce snack 2 hours later. My energy remains good and my blood glucose readings are stable and normal.
- Pizza made with white sauce, some meat and hard cheese along with a salad of veggies and greens provides a good dinner or lunch.
- At dinner I have chicken, fish or beef with veggies and a small portion of potato, rice or pasta. I fix a cream sauce using cream and butter to put over the protein and veggies, just a small amount is necessary. That can keep me stabilized for 2-4 hours depending how active I am in the evening.
- When I have a craving for sweets I have real ice cream, a chocolate, or butter cookie. These have a high ratio of fat to sugar so my gut tolerates the sugar a little better. I also eat the sweets after a meal so my gut is already set with good foods. Soft drinks, cakes and frosting, candy without fat will set my blood glucose dropping quickly and radically. My personality goes down the toilet too.

Self Care for Reactive Hypoglycemia Tendencies

- Blood glucose testing multiple times/day
- Nutritional changes:
  - small meals every 2 hours
  - fat/protein to carbohydrate ratio increased
  - zone diet: 40% carbohydrate, 30% protein, 30% fat
  - fat/protein at breakfast to set the enteric brake
  - refined sugars, fruit juice, white flour eliminated
  - vitamin/mineral boosters
    - chromium picolinate 300-600 mcg
    - vitamin B complex 50-100 mg
    - coenzyme Q 25-50 mg
    - zinc 50 mg
  - amino acid complex
  - herb booster
    - bilberry
    - wild yam

In comparing General Hypoglycemic Tendencies with Reactive Hypoglycemic Tendencies it is noted that both cases exhibit imbalance between insulin and glucose in the bloodstream. In the case of General Hypoglycemic Tendencies, increased complex carbohydrate intake is a major factor in stimulating the appropriate insulin-glucose ratio in the bloodstream. In the case of Reactive Hypoglycemic Tendencies, an increased protein and fat ratio to carbohydrates is a major factor in balancing the insulin-glucose ratio in the bloodstream. Each individual must use trial and error to determine his/her individual needs.

Hypothyroid Tendencies

Tyrosine and iodine are components necessary to form thyroxine, the thyroid hormone. If the amino acid tyrosine is low it may cause hypothyroid tendencies in FMS individuals. Slagle describes using tyrosine and iodine to successfully treat hypothyroid tendencies.

Individuals with cell level hypothyroid tendency type symptoms may be helped by taking 2000-3000 mg Kelp daily for iodine and L-Tyrosine 500 mg 2 times daily for essential amino acid with water or juice, not with milk or other protein. For better absorption take the tyrosine with 50 mg B6 and 100 mg vitamin C. The tyrosine and iodine combine to form the active thyroid hormone T3.

Food sources of tyrosine include almonds, avocados, bananas, dairy products, lima beans, pumpkin seed and sesame seeds. Supplements of L tyrosine should be taken at bedtime or with a carbohydrate meal so it does not competing for absorption with other amino acids.

Adding phytoestrogen and/or progesterone in cream or food form may improve the symptoms of cell level hypothyroid tendency in individuals with fibromyalgia and reproductive hormonal dysfunction.

Fatty acids are also needed by the thyroid system to function effectively. Fatty acids are the building blocks of some messenger chemicals and come from the breakdown of fats and oils. Essential fatty acids (EFAs) cannot be produced in the body and must be supplied through the diet and broken down into fatty acid form in the gut. Fatty acids are needed for rebuilding and producing all cells in the body. Sources of essential fatty acids include fish oils, flaxseeds and flaxseed oil, grape seed oil and primrose oil. Amounts will vary depending on the supplement.

Vitamin B complex including Vitamin B12 is essential for cellular oxygenation and energy production. It is also needed for proper digestion of proteins into amino acids and fats into fatty acids. Fifty to 100 mg of vitamin B complex and 15-45 mg of vitamin B12 may be beneficial in facilitating cell metabolism and reducing "hypothyroid" symptoms.

The stomach digests apples and other fruits converting the fruit into malic acid along with other components. Malic acid is an essential acid for energy or ATP production at the cell level. Malic acid has the ability to increase utilization of needed substances including sugars for ATP production even under low oxygen conditions. It is a part of the efficient metabolism process in every body cell. Suggested malic acid intake is 1200-1400 mg/day.

The stomach and small intestine digests green leafy vegetables, legumes and nuts to obtain magnesium. Magnesium is the fourth most abundant mineral in the body. It is the number one stress mineral. ATP production is dependent on adequate magnesium levels at the cellular level. Magnesium facilitates enzyme function for metabolic action in each cell. It lights the spark (the enzyme) that lights the fire or starts the motor (metabolism) of each cell. It facilitates ATP energy into physical and mental function. Suggested magnesium intake is 500-800 mg/day.

Fluoride and chlorine are chemically related to iodine. These chemicals interfere with the body's ability to absorb iodine from food. They can block iodine receptors in the thyroid gland resulting in reduced iodine available in the thyroid and thus reduced iodine combined with tyrosine to form T4. Avoiding chlorinated water, and fluoride toothpastes, may be of help in decreasing FMS symptoms.

Self Care for Hypothyroid Tendencies

- Basal body temperature testing
- Nutritional changes:
  - kelp 1000-3000 mg
  - amino acids – L-tyrosine 1000 mg
  - vitamin B12 15-45 mg
  - vitamin B6 50 mg
  - magnesium 400-600 mg
  - essential fatty acids
  - avoid chlorine and fluoride
- Phytoestrogen and progesterone

Neurally Mediated Hypotension Tendencies

Initial treatment for NMH tendencies involves a self care routine. If the self care routine is not adequate then the tilt test is performed and specific medications can be prescribed.

Salt (NACL)

The first step in self care for NMH is to salt all foods, salt during cooking, bullion cubes in gravies and soups and salt tablets if exercising or perspiring. If these strategies do not increase salt levels and decrease symptoms, the tests can be completed and medication prescribed.

Accentuate the Positive, Eliminate the Negative
in the Enteric Nervous System (ENS)

The second step in self care for NMH is to assist the ENS in normal function. The ENS produces important chemical messengers that affect blood pressure and heart rate. These chemical messengers are formed from amino acid necklaces present in the gut therefore producing normal levels of these amino acid necklaces is essential. Increasing protein and/or amino acid intake can be beneficial. A variety of meat and fish are needed because each contains different levels of the various amino acids. Another way to obtain the needed amino acids is through supplements containing amino acids with complementing vitamins and minerals.

Some food products stabilize and are beneficial to ENS production of chemical messengers that affect heart rate and blood pressure. Turkey contains high levels of tryptophan which is the precursor to serotonin so turkey will likely stimulate the ENS in a positive way. Milk products also contain tryptophan and can be useful in facilitating sleep and normalizing body functions. Applesauce, bananas, and rice have been known by every mother whose child has diarrhea to quiet the enteric system.When the ENS is sluggish, foods containing caffeine, spices like red pepper, and roughage can stimulate peristaltic action. Small amounts of these foods go a long way.

Sugars

Sugar (glucose) in the small intestine stimulates enteric nerve activity to gut and pancreas so insulin and glucose are released excessively. The result can be low blood sugar levels with symptoms being incoordination, weakness, confusion, and agitation. Sugars ingested by a sugar sensitive individual with CPP can set off a cascade of events initiated by the enteric nervous system. Using the same rationale, eliminating simple sugars and consuming complex carbohydrates with fats and protein could potentially prevent the hypersensitive reaction. The symptoms of fatigue, weakness, confusion, and personality change can be significantly decreased or eliminated.

Fats

Fats taken into the digestive system slow intestinal peristalsis. In the most drastic situation the enteric brake stops peristalsis all together until the fats are broken down by the bile salts into smaller molecules. Therefore fat intake can be used as an inhibitor of enteric nervous system activation of peristalsis. At the same time fat's quieting inhibitory effect on the enteric nervous system affects many other organ systems, i.e. bladder, uterus, heart, and has a quieting affect on them too.

Proteins

Proteins taken into the digestive system take longer for the enteric nervous system to break down than sugars and carbohydrates. The proteins tend to slow the enteric system's action. So a relatively high protein intake may help an individual with high resting heart rate and low blood pressure. The quieting affect of protein is not as great as the quieting affect of fat.

Eliminate Food Sensitivity

Eliminating food products that destabilize the ENS improves chemical messenger production and function. Elimination of nicotine, caffeine and simple sugars can be helpful. Hypersensitivity to certain foods can play a role in ENS dysfunction. When bloating, gas, alternating diarrhea and constipation is present, food hypersensitivity may play a role in NMH tendencies. Lactose intolerance is the sensitivity to milk products. Wheat intolerance is the sensitivity to breads, pastas, and cereals containing wheat. Even the thickening in gravies and stews or soups may contain wheat. Monosodium glutamate (MSG) intolerance is the sensitivity to an additive found in many prepared foods. The symptoms are very similar to NMH tendencies.

Dehydration

Dehydration is a major factor in gut dysfunction, causing constipation, fecal impaction and inflammation. Water in adequate amounts is a stimulus to gut peristalsis. Drinking 6-8 glasses of noncaffeinated fluid is the general recommendation. Individuals will state that they drink 6-8 glasses of fluid per day but if the majority of that is caffeinated or alcohol, both diuretics, the result is dehydration.

Monitor Magnesium Levels

Individuals with low blood pressure need to monitor the amount of magnesium they take since magnesium is an effective smooth muscle relaxant. That means high levels of magnesium could potentially lower blood pressure even more. Since magnesium is low in some individuals with CPP there is a tendency to supplement at high levels. For the individual with CPP and low blood pressure, moderate levels of magnesium supplementation, 300-400 mg/day, is more often recommended. Blood pressure should be monitored when adding magnesium.

Self Care for Neurally Mediated Hypotension Tendencies

- Blood pressure and heart rate monitoring
- Nutritional changes:
  - salt, sodium chloride increase
  - magnesium levels monitored
  - caffeine, refined sugars, alcohol eliminated
  - amino acid complex increase
  - gut (enteric) normalizing foods
    - turkey, rice, applesauce, bananas
  - herb: licorice
- Pelvic vericosity drainage
  - hips higher than heart
- Essential oils
  - teas: peppermint, chamomile
  - external: angelica, balm, bergamot, clary, lavendar, mint, neroli

Reproductive Hormone Deregulation Tendencies

Supplementing with phytoestrogens and/or progesterones in food or cream form or using hormone replacement therapy on a temporary or permanent basis may assist the organ systems in balanced function. Self care treatment can include using phytoestrogen and phytoprogesterone on a cyclical basis. Over the counter creams can be used. Phytoestrogens are available in foods such as soy, flax seed, and green tea. Many vegetables have natural estrogen components- green beans, carrots, peas, and beets are a few. Some fruits have estrogen components also – these include cherries, apples and rhubarb. Phytoprogesterones are in soybeans and yams. Prescription hormone replacement therapy is also available. In a clinical trial, pain and fatigue, bowel, bladder and menstrual cycle dysfunction improved in a small group of women who used phytoestrogen and progesterone during the winter and spring months.

Relaxin is available in nonprescription form as a nutritional supplement.

Oxytocin is available in prescription form only.

DHEA is available in prescription or nonprescription forms. It also can be restored and maintained by joy, sexual activity, physical exercise, positive thinking and sunshine. Vitamin C (2000 mg/day) and Methyl Sulfonyl Methane (1000 mg/day) may be of benefit in raising the DHEA levels. Yams, used in manufacturing DHEA, cannot be used by the body to convert to DHEA. Shealy has found topical progesterone cream (UPS grade 3%), 1/4 teaspoon twice daily has sometimes facilitated increased DHEA levels. In a study by Meely adding 50mg of DHEA daily improved reproductive hormone levels, skin integrity, energy levels and mood stability.

Self Care for Reproductive Hormone Dysfunction Tendencies

- Hormonal tests and monthly symptom diary
- Nutritional changes:
  - estrogen/progesterone rich foods
    - soy, flax seed, green tea
  - caffeine, refined sugars eliminated
  - vitamin C 250-1000 mg
- Nonprescriptive creams or supplements:
  - phytoestrogen cream
  - phytoprogesterone cream
  - DHEA
  - phytoestrogen/progesterone supplements
- Fun, laughter, joy

Bowel Program

Healthy bowel function is essential to decrease CPP. Constipation, irritable bowel syndrome, diarrhea, or flatulence can all increase discomfort and pain in the pelvic region. A healthy bowel function is defined as bowel movements 3 times per week of soft-formed consistency that are eliminated without straining.

A bowel program for constipation includes:

- 6-8 glasses of fluid daily
- Eliminate caffeine and alcohol
- Fruits and vegetables 5-6 per day
  - One at breakfast
  - Two at lunch and dinner
- Bran or flaxseed and yogurt at breakfast
  - 1-2 teaspoons bran or 1-2 tablespoons flaxseed
  - 4-6 oz. yogurt
- Magnesium 250-500 mg
  Vitamin C 250-1000 mg (not recommended if renal failure or interstitial cystitis so check with physician before using)
- Core PMFF exercises
- Self massage with Phoenix Massage Oil or olive oil
  - Clockwise circular massage from lower right abdomen up, across, and down left lower abdomen
  - Daily before arising
  - Follow with drinking 2 cups of warm water

Advanced Acupressure/Massage Techniques

As described in the Basic Self Care Techniques, acupressure applied for 7-8 seconds to appropriate tender points can be beneficial in relieving CPP. Acupressure points in the abdomen, groin, leg, low back and sacral areas are accessible for external surface pressure. (Figure 49)

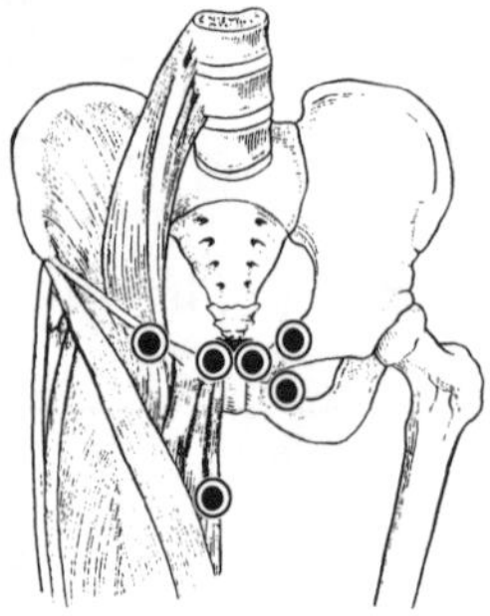

Advanced acupressure techniques include more specific points in the abdomen and groin to target specific muscles. Additionally advanced techniques include treatment of

Figure 49
External Tender Points

tender or trigger points internally- accessible through the vaginal wall. The technique is similar to external acupressure – firm but gentle pressure for 7-8 seconds over the tender or trigger point. (Figure 50)

Technique:

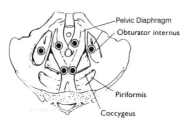

- Pelvic Diaphragm
- Obturator internus
- Piriformis
- Coccygeus

Figure 50
Internal Tender Points

- Locate the tender point or trigger point through palpation.
- Maintain direct pressure over the point for 7-8 seconds with the muscle and fascia in a slack position. Use diaphragmatic breathing for improved release.
- Repeat 3-4 times throughout the day.

Treat the Feet-Improve Chronic Pelvic Pain

The Innervation Is The Same

The foot is connected with CPP through common nerve innervation, fascial/ligamentous planes and functional movements such as ambulation. The intrinsic foot muscles function in coordination with pelvic muscle function via striated muscle innervation from sacral nerve roots 2-5. These nerve roots are responsible for sensory and motor innervation of levator ani, urogenital diaphragm, and obturator internus and the foot intrinsic muscles. The human embryo has a tail that is reabsorbed during weeks 5 and 6 of gestation. During the caudal regression process of the tail asymmetrical and symmetrical neuronal loss may occur that affects sacral roots 2-5. Motor and/or sensory deficits in the feet occur simultaneously with pelvic muscle dysfunction and sensory loss as described by Galloway. In theory, strengthening foot musculature can improve pelvic pain and pelvic muscle function. Sensory stimulation of the feet can improve pain and function within the pelvis. Ambulation has the potential to improve CPP and PMFF function.

The Foot is Connected to the Leg Bone...
To the Pelvis...

The chain of fascia and ligaments extending from the foot to the lumbo-pelvic region is continuous such that distal movements of the lower leg and foot can assist in stability of the pelvis. The pelvic diaphragm connects to the obturator internus to the sacrotuberous and sacrospinous ligaments that interconnect with the biceps femoris which attaches to the head of the fibula and fascial planes which interconnect with the peroneals, navicular and fifth metatarsal bones of the feet. Plantar flexion and dorsiflexion and inversion sends forces through fascial interconnections to stabilize the sacrum. That improves lumbo-sacral stability during gait and upper extremity activities.

Foot Massage

Foot massage stimulates sacral nerves that innervate the feet and pelvic region. This is termed retrograde stimulation of pelvic muscles and organs. Massage the plantar aspect of the foot in a clockwise circular fashion using the knuckles. Begin at the heel, moving up the longitudinal arch to the transverse arch. Massage across the transverse arch, then down the lateral border to the heel, then up the center of the sole of the foot. Repeat 4-5 times. (Figure 51)

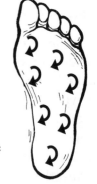

Massage each toe, grasping it and wringer-washing it gently from base to tip. Then massage between each toe with a finger.

Use Phoenix Massage Oil or olive oil to moisturize the feet and decrease pain when doing massage.

Figure 51: Foot Massage

Foot Exercises

Foot exercises stimulate sacral nerve fibers in similar fashion to foot massage. Perform exercises one foot at a time, 10-12 slow repetitions, with diaphragmatic breathing. (Figure 52)

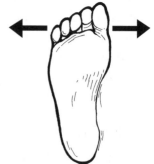

Dorsiflexion/plantarflexion
Toe curls/toe straightening
Toe spreading/toe closing
Clockwise foot circles

Figure 52: Foot Exercise

Walking

Wearing comfortable supportive shoes, walk 20-30 minutes daily. If there is significant foot dysfunction or gait deviation foot orthotics or special exercises are recommended.

Oils and Creams

Plant oils have been used for many centuries to improve health and treat illness. Oil is absorbed by the skin and can reach other organs and tissues through the connective tissue and the lymphatic and circulatory systems. In the earliest healing practices plants were utilized by eating the raw leaves, berries, or bark. Later, burning or cooking the plant parts expanded the healing arts. Two to three thousand years before Christ the Romans, Indians, and Chinese were using plant oils for medicinal and religious purposes. The Rigveda of India states "...come, you wise plants, heal this patient for me." The Romans used plants in the form of pills, powders, suppositories, purees, ointments and pastes for external use. Ancient Greeks used plants and flowers for medicinal and cosmetic purposes. Hippocrates cited medicinal plants and stated, "Let your medicine be your food and your food be your medicine". Avicenna, the great Arab physician, describes over 800 plants and their effects on the human body. He also is credited with perfecting the process of distilling plants into essential oils. In more modern times, a French chemist Dr. Rene-Maurice Gattefosse coined the term aromatherapy and a French physician Dr. Jean Valnet used essential oils in treating war injuries during WWII to disinfect and heal. British and Italian scientists published research about medicinal qualities of essential oils in the 1920s and 30s.

Essential oils come from plant parts. The oil is located in or on the surface of the plant tissue in the form of tiny sacs or globules. A familiar fruit, the orange, has its oil in the rind that is peeled to arrive at the fruit. The functions of essential oils for the plant are to ward off harmful insects, attract beneficial ones, protect the plant from bacteria or fungal infections, and communicate to the rest of the plant and animal world.

The distillation method is much like distilling whiskey. Small amounts of the desired plant and water are placed in a container that is heated. The oil droplets are carried by steam into a tube cooled by cold water that carries the oil droplets into another container. The second container is filled with water. The oil separates from the water. In most cases it rises to the top, being lighter than water. In a few cases the oil falls to the bottom, the oil being heavier than water. In either case, it can be collected for use as essential oil.

Oils and creams have the potential to relieve pelvic pain. Phoenix Massage Oil used on the lower abdomen, low back and inner thighs has been beneficial for some individuals with CPP. It can increase circulation, decrease muscle spasm, and decrease congestion.

The most common oil to use in the vulva area is extra virgin olive oil. It has been used through the centuries as soothing, healing oil. It can be applied with fingertips in a gentle fashion.

Estrogen/progesterone cream applied intravaginally can increase lubrication and decrease pain. Phytoestrogen or progesterone cream applied to the lower abdomen or inner thighs can have the same affect.

Nitroglycerin cream is sometimes used when other trials have been ineffective. It is applied to the vulvar area.

Modalities

Electrical Stimulation

Equipment using electrical current may assist in pain control. Modalities that can be helpful include high voltage galvanic stimulation, neuromuscular electrical stimulation, transcutaneous electrical stimulation, interferential current stimulation, and microamperage. Electrical stimulation in the form of high voltage galvanic stimulation or interferential current stimulation is delivered through moist pads over muscle areas which are connected to a piece of equipment via wires. The electric stimulation causes pulsation and a "buzzing" may be felt during the treatment.

Electrical current in the various forms increases circulation and facilitates muscle relaxation as well as decreases pain and spasm. Contraindications include a heart pacemaker, pregnancy, cancer, severe musculoskeletal lesions, or active inflammation or infection. It can be appropriate for general pelvic pain syndromes including endometriosis, dysmenorrhea, pelvic inflammatory disease, coccygodynia, vulvodynia, perineal pain, and levator ani syndrome.

Parameters: High voltage galvanic stimulation is often effective at 50-100 volts, 80 pulses per second, negative polarity, 2.5 seconds reciprocal for 20 minutes. Interferential current stimulation is effective for chronic pain at 0-10 Hz, 15 sec. scan time, fast 90° vector auto intensity 0, carrier frequency 5 KHz, 20 minutes.

Transcutaneous electrical stimulation can be used in the conventional method at 60-100 Hz or in the acupuncture method at 2-10 Hz, 100-250 microseconds.

Neuromuscular electrical stimulation can be used at 100 Hz, 250-400 microseconds.

Microamperage is often effective in the same areas at .5 uv for 20 minutes using silver-silver chloride electrodes.

Electrode Placement: Electrode placements are usually in proximity to target nerves and muscles. Effective placements include bilateral sacrum and bilateral ischial tuberosity or bilateral ischial tuberosities and bilateral suprapubic region. If pain is primarily in the abdominal region placement can be bilateral upper and lower abdominal areas. Placing the large dispersive pad over the lower abdomen and the smaller pads over the lumbar paraspinals and sacral area is effective in treating deep muscles such as the iliopsoas. Placing two pads in the lumbo sacral area and two small pads suprapubically in a pattern is effective in treating the pelvic muscles.

Electrical stimulation can be used with internal vaginal or anal probes. Intravaginal electrical stimulation to inhibit pain uses 5-20 Hz, 100-1000 msec duration, 1:2 work/rest cycle, 15-30 minutes, symmetrical or asymmetrical, 1-2 times per day. Turn the intensity up gradually to accommodate the new feeling. It should not be painful but instead a perceptible, comfortable feeling.

Ultrasound

Ultrasound has the potential to decrease muscle spasm and pain, increase blood flow to the affected region, and soften connective scar tissue. Contraindications include infection, pregnancy, cancer, vascular disease, and decreased sensation. It is not recommended to use ultrasound over ovaries. It can be appropriate for treating vaginisimus, pelvic muscle pain, coccygodynia, and hemorrhoids.

Parameters: For trigger points use .5 w/cm² in a slow circle. For piriformis syndrome or deep pelvic muscle spasm/pain use 1.75 w/cm². For levator ani syndrome use 1-2.5 w/cm² around the anus for 3-5 minutes. For perineal pain use 1.5 w/cm² over a water or gel condom or with the perineal area submerged in water.

Myofascial Release

Myofascial release techniques incorporate three-dimensional stretching and inhibition techniques for balancing biomechanical and neurological dysfunctions of the musculoskeletal system. Muscle and fascia have inherent motion and visco-elastic properties. Muscle and fascial dysfunction is exhibited as fascial resistance to voluntary, passive or inherent motion.

Myofascial release techniques include direct and indirect approaches to unwinding tissue tension. In the direct approach, pressure on tissues follows the direction of ease. In the indirect approach pressure on tissues is toward the direction of increased tension. The desired result is release of tissue tension – a softening. (Figure 53)

The application of myofascial release techniques for CPP includes:

■ Contacting tissue surface with hand surface – the treatment hand is in contact with the tissues to be treated. This involves a molding and conformation of the treating hand to the treating surface.

■ Identifying tissue quality, tension, tone, temperature, moisture, texture using the treatment hand contact.

■ Facilitating active, passive and inherent tissue mobility with pressure from the treatment hand. Follow into the direction of ease (direct) or resistance (indirect). Hold at the balance point or barrier (still point). Feel the release and follow the release phenomena. Repeat until there is a three-dimensional balance.

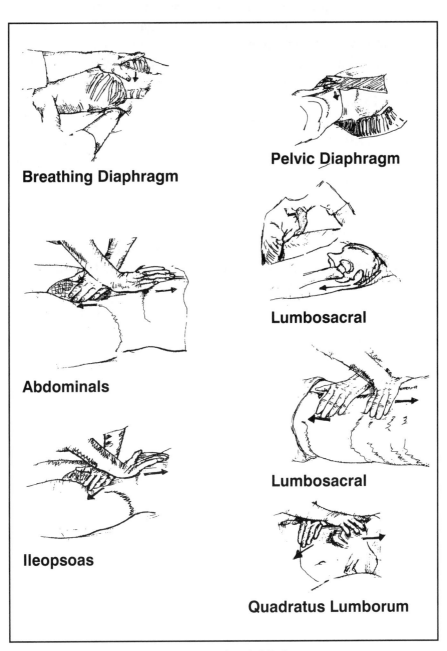

Breathing Diaphragm

Pelvic Diaphragm

Abdominals

Lumbosacral

Ileopsoas

Lumbosacral

Quadratus Lumborum

Figure 53: Myofascial Release

Visceral Mobilization

Visceral mobilization techniques therapeutically move organs to restore their inherent motion. Abdominal organs exhibit active and passive motion. Active motion is termed organ mobility and occurs in response to stimulation by the somatic nervous system or the breathing diaphragm. Passive motion is termed organ motility and is innate and intrinsic. Each organ has its own frequency and amplitude of motion. When the frequency or amplitude of an organ is altered illness occurs according to Barral. Chronic pelvic pain is often seen in conjunction with limitations of urogenital motility or mobility. Facilitating a return to normal motion may improve the symptoms of CPP. (Figure 54)

The application of visceral techniques include:

- Listening to determine the location of the organ restriction. "Listening" is with hands located over the area and feeling the passive inherent motions. The hand attracts body motion to it. The hand is drawn to the area of dysfunction.

- Testing for mobility and motility of the urogenital organs.

- Treating for visceral mobility and motility by following the rhythmical motion of organs. Accentuating the part of the rhythmical cycle with the greater amplitude and gently stretching the organ motion are beneficial.

Therapeutic Intervention Strategies Related to Posttraumatic Stress Disorder (PTSD)

Therapeutic intervention strategies in relation to PTSD involves the usual physical and functional goals as well as psychosocial goals. The goals for a clinician while interacting with an individual experiencing PTSD include:

- Acknowledge and manage his/her own feelings about PTSD
- Build trust without becoming "hooked" by the individual's issues
- Define and maintain appropriate boundaries
- Develop effective physical intervention strategies

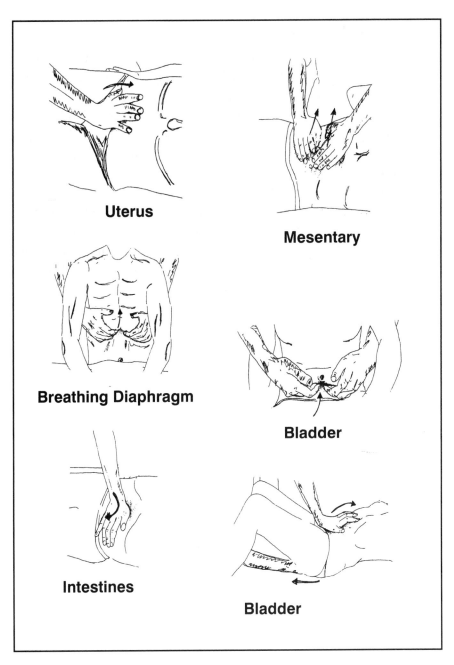

Uterus

Mesentary

Breathing Diaphragm

Bladder

Intestines

Bladder

Figure 54: Visceral Mobilization

Coping behaviors in PTSD can include dissociative, sexualized, physiologic defense, cognitive defense, and internal control behaviors.

Dissociative Behavior

In dissociative behavior, touch may recreate the abuse stimulus which sets off the body separation from the mind. The individual is not able to give accurate information about his physical being because the message system between the body and mind is blocked. The mind is not receiving accurate information about the body. The individual is unable to have internal controls for exercise duration or intensity when there is no feedback to the mind about pain, fatigue or energy level.

Therapeutic intervention instruction needs to be consistent with words, format, and behavior at each session. Explain the anatomy, the desired activity and the expected result clearly and simply. Obtain permission for each new step, give choices and let the individual make the decisions. Empower the individual. Always observe body language and compare with the verbal information the client gives. The individual with PTSD needs no distractions for learning to occur. The environment must be quiet and safe.

Sexualized Behavior

In sexualized behavior the individual may exhibit inappropriate sexual behavior or misinterpret the clinician's behavior as being sexually attracting. Off hand jokes or remarks of a sexual nature may be interpreted as attraction by the client. Friendship or social interaction outside the therapy setting may be interpreted as an intimate message.

The clinician can initially clearly define herself as a helping professional rather than as a friend. Always have eye contact while working with the individual. Be calm, respond in a professional manner to any overt sexual behavior. Use objective directions as to what is necessary for you to be able to interact effectively in a therapeutic environment.

Physiologic Defense Behavior

In physiologic defense behavior the individual exhibits inaccurate perception to sensory input. For example there can be hypersensitivity to touch or movement. There may be numbness in certain body parts. In either instance there is inaccurate feedback between the body and mind.

The clinician initially needs to develop activities for body and mind connections. Association techniques can include use of biofeedback EMG using visual feedback about muscle activity at rest and during physical exertion. Association techniques can include perceiving the color, texture, and temperature of each body part. External measurement tools such as EMG and temperature can help determine appropriate levels of exercise when the individual is unable to limit activities based on accurate internal feedback.

Begin by instructing the individual with releasing and relaxing, then describing how that released muscle tone feels. Begin with breathing and feeling the inhale and exhale. Then describe the feeling of each breath. Begin with perceiving left and right hand temperature, then learn to warm the hands. When those exercises have become easy it is possible to progress to slow, easy, minimal levels of exercise, floating through the small movements as slowly and smoothly as possible while maintaining a regular breathing pattern.

In the home environment begin with the basic self care loop which includes sleep protocol, nutrition, and positive self statements.

Cognitive Defense Behavior

In cognitive defense behavior the individual exhibits low self esteem, poor self care and sometimes self abuse. This leads to problems carrying out a therapy program. The individual cannot carry through with a home program because she feels such hate or shame. The feeling of shame is constant and infects all daily life accomplishments.

The individual feels unworthy of success so he or she may sabotage physical activities. She feels unworthy of the effort it takes to do exercise consistently. The individual may use therapy tools for self abuse.

The clinician's offhand remarks about weakness, softness, or anything remotely negative or less than perfect may be amplified by the individual, taken as "bad" which can bring out shame and powerlessness. Clinician's comments such as "why didn't you......" bring on the shame feelings. The denial of stated client feelings, such as "No, you don't feel that way...." or "That's no way to feel....." brings on the shame feelings. Instead of asking "why?" which brings on increased shame, ask "could you tell me a little more about that?"

The clinician can give consistent affirmations at appropriate developmental levels. During treatment active listening and eye contact help to validate the client and empower the individual to positive action. The clinician can direct small steps for self care that are not overwhelming and actively involve the individual in decision making.

Internal Control – Limit Setting Behavior

In internal control-limit setting behavior the individual exhibits physical disorientation, an inability to set internal limits and an inability to carry through with self care in any consistent manner. Nutrition, exercise and work limits are often erratic and eccentric, serving from one extreme to another. The individual either overdoes an activity or does nothing. Clinicians can encourage and help to structure self care strategies with a balance of work and rest, to develop cycles of sleep, nutrition, exercise, work and leisure. The role of the clinician is to tailor pacing of exercise, activities of daily living, and work to the needs of the individual as a whole and integrated person. Sometimes that involves eliminating activities or going back to a blank slate and then adding one or two new steps carried out consistently for a period of time before adding another activity. Other times changing one activity in the daily life of the individual will be the best approach to developing internal control and limit setting behavior. Still other times it means interjecting a new behavior multiple times into the day to reconnect body and mind and interrupt running on automatic pilot. In each of these cases the therapist helps the individual to learn new skills as a substitute for inappropriate ones.

Guidelines for Treatment

The following are general guidelines for developing effective therapeutic interventions when PTSD is a factor.

1. Stop at each step, explain and obtain permission for the next step.

2. Check that the individual is staying with his/her body during treatment.

3. If the individual exhibits self defeating behaviors address them

before expecting progress in the therapy program.

4. Start with concreteness, i.e.. EMG to develop trust and interest. The individual is very curious and interested at a conscious and unconscious level.

5. Inform the individual of options for treatment and let her/him choose the next step.

6. Ask how the individual best learns, through sight, verbage, demonstration. Then use that mode in teaching.

7. Use a private room with definite boundaries such as doors being closed.

8. Define the boundaries of treatment – the therapist is the guide, the individual is the empowered leader to heal.

9. Monitor home program follow-through, one self-care priority at a time.

10. Never shame the individual. "Why didn't you?" "No, you shouldn't feel this way."

11. Be cautious about setting up unrealistic treatment goals that then end in failure and shame for the individual.

12. Use constant affirmations such as "I'm glad you are here." "I trust you to take care of yourself." "I know you had good reasons for your actions." "I know you did the best thing for you at the time."

13. Be aware the individual will test you to see if you are really listening, to see if you really care, to see if you are human, to see if you are giving power and control back to them with boundaries or just pretending.

14. Exhibit compassion not loving. Compassion is deep affection, understanding and gentleness.

15. When talking to the individual always face him/her. Turning away indicates abandonment.

16. Many individuals are compartmentalized. Breathing and talking at the same time will be difficult. Breathing and eating may not

be possible. Stress is stored and does not move up and out. So outline one activity at a time beginning with the basics of breathing, talking and eating.

17. Believe healing is possible.

18. Be willing to witness emotional pain with empathy not pity.

19 Be willing to believe the unbelievable.

20 Examine your own attitudes. If you have abuse issues in your background that have not been dealt with do not attempt to take on an individual with those issues. Refer them to someone else.

Chapter 17

Treatment Suggestions by Subcategory

The following subcategory treatment suggestions are intended for use after the self-care management strategies in chapter 15 have been completed. Identifying your subcategory and following these treatment protocols is an important part of treatment but will only be effective when used in conjunction with general self-care strategies.

Levator Ani Syndrome

- PMFF electrical stimulation
- Bowel program
- Advanced PMFF exercise
- Acupressure
- Pelvic warming

Piriformis Syndrome

- Advanced PMFF exercise-adductor phase
- Pelvic warming

Coccygodynia

- PMFF electrical stimulation
- Bowel program
- Advanced PMFF exercise-adductor phase
- Acupressure
- Pelvic warming

Vaginisimus

- Hot shower/bath
- P.Q. during penetration
- Basic and advanced PMFF exercises
- Estrogen and testosterone cream
- Visceral motility
- Nitroglycerine cream
- Vaginal dilators
- Massage: desensitizing and trigger point

Dyspareunia

- Hot shower/bath
- P.Q. during penetration
- Basic and advanced PMFF exercises
- Estrogen and testosterone cream
- Visceral motility
- Nitroglycerine cream
- Vaginal dilators
- Massage: desensitizing and trigger point

Proctalgia Fugax

- Anal electrical stimulation
- Bowel program
- Advanced PMFF exercise-adductor phase
- Acupressure
- Pelvic warming

Vulvar Vestibulitis – Vulvodynia

- Extra virgin olive oil
- Estrogen and testosterone cream
- Nitroglycerin cream
- Dietary changes
- Desensitizing massage

Pudendal Neuralgia

- Alternate ice and heat
- Stretches
- Deep massage

Pelvic Muscle Relaxation Syndromes

- Hip elevation with PMFF exercises
- Hip elevation during rest periods
- Avoid heavy lifting
- Estrogen and progesterone cream

Urological Syndromes

- Vapocoolant spray and heat
- Acupressure
- Essential oil massage externally
- High voltage galvanic stimulation externally

Interstitial Cystitis

- Vaginal electrical stimulation
- Pelvic warming
- Vapocoolant spray and heat
- Essential oil massage externally
- Visceral motility

Prostatitis

- Vapocoolant spray and heat
- Accupressure
- Essential oil massage externally
- High voltage galvanic stimulation externally
- Pelvic warming

Neurally Mediated Hypotension - Pelvic Congestion

- Dietary salt
- Hip elevation with PMFF exercises
- Elevated bed bottom
- Essential oil massage externally
- Pool exercises
- Visceral motility

Post Traumatic Stress Disorder

- Therapeutic ball activities
- Pelvic warming
- Acupressure
- Foot massage
- Essential oil massage
- Advanced P.Q. - imagine space

References

Chapter One, Two, Three

Bass E. *The Courage to Heal: A Guide to Women Survivors of Childhood Sexual Abuse.* New York: Harper & Row, 1988.

Howard F. *Pelvic Pain: Diagnosis and Management.* New York: Lippincott Williams & Wilkins, 2000.

Hulme J. *Fibromyalgia: A Handbook For Self Care & Treatment.* 3rd Edition. Missoula, MT: Phoenix Pub., 1999

Lee D. *The Pelvic Girdle: An Approach to the Examination and Treatment of the Lumbo-Pelvic-Hip Region,* New York, NY: Churchill Livingstone; 1999.

Palter S ed. *Chronic Pelvic Pain. Intertility and Reproductive Medicine Clinics of North America.* Philadelphia: W.B. Saunders, 1999.

Rocker I ed. *Pelvic Pain in Women: Diagnosis and Management.* New Yorrk: Springer-Verlag, 1989.

Scully R, Barnes M. *Physical Therapy.* New York, NY: Lippincott Co; 1989.

Simons DG, Travell JG, Simons LS. *Myofascial Pain and Dysfunction: Thr Trigger Point Manual Vol. 2,* 2nd ed. Baltimore: Williams and Wilkins, 1999.

Steege J, Metzger D, Levy B. *Chronic Pelvic Pain: An Integrated Approach.* Philadelphia: W.R. Saunders, 1998.

Chapter Four

Childre D et. al. *The Heartmath Solution.* San Francisco: HarperCollins, 1999.

Cutler W, Garcia C. *Menopause A Guide for Women and the Men Who Love Them* (revised). New York: WW Norton & Co, 1992.

Fried R. *The Hyperventilation Syndrome: Research and Clinical Treatment.* Baltimore: John Hopkins University Press, 1987.

Gershon M. *The Second Brain,* New York: HarperCollins, 1998.

Goldstein J et. al. *Betrayal of the Brain: The Neurologic Basis of Chronic Fatigue Syndrome, Fibromyalgia Syndrome and Related Neural Network Disorders.* Binghampton, NY: Haworth Press, 1996.

Griep EN et. al. Altered reactivity of the HPA axis in the primary fibromyalgia syndrome. *Jrnl of Rheum* 20:469-474, 1993.

Hendricks G. *Conscious Breathing.* New York: Bantam Books, 1995.

Ornish D. *Love and Survival The Scientific Basis for the Healing Power of Intimacy.* New York: HarperCollins, 1997.

Pellegrino MJ et. al. Familial occurrence of primary fibromyalgia. *Arch Phys Med Rehabil* 70:61-63, 1989.

Pert C. *Molecules of Emotion. The Science Behind Mind-Body Medicine.* New York: Simon & Schuster, 1997.

Slagle P. *The Way Up From Down.* New York: Random House, 1987.

Teitelbaum J. *From Fatigued to Fantastic A Manual for Moving Beyond Chronic Fatigue and Fibromyalgia.* Garden City Park, NY: Avery Publishing, 1996.

Yunus, MB et. al. A study of multicase families with fibromyalgia with HLA typing. *Arthritis Rheum* 35:S285, 1992.

Chapter Five

Howard F. *Pelvic Pain: Diagnosis and Management.* New York: Lippincott Williams & Wilkins, 2000.

Simons DG, Travell JG, Simons LS. *Myofascial Pain and Dysfunction: Thr Trigger Point Manual* Vol. 2, 2nd ed. Baltimore: Williams and Wilkins, 1999.

Chapter Six

Hulme J. *Beyond Kegels: Fabulous Four Exercises to Prevent and Treat Incontinence.* Missoula, Mont: Phoenix Publishing; 1997.

Chapter Seven

Hulme J. *Beyond Kegels Book II: A Clinicians Guide to Treatment Algorithms and Special Populations.* Missoula Mont: Phoenix Publishing; 1998.

Chapter Eight

Galloway N. The Challenge of a Painful Bladder. In: Conner WH, ed. *Mediguide to Urology,* New York, NY: Lawrence DellaCarte Publishing, 1994.

Hodges PW. Richardson CA. Inefficient muscular stabilization of the lumbar spine associated with low back pain: a motor control evaluation of transverses abdominis. *Spine,* 1996:21(22); 2640-2650.

Mooney V. *Sacroiliac Joint Dysfunction: Movement, Stability and Low Back Pain.* Edinburgh, Scotland: Churchill Livingstone; 1997.

Richardson C, Jull G, Hodges P, Hides J. *Therapeutic Exercise for Spinal Segmental Stabilization in Low Back Pain.* New York: Churchill Livingston, 1999.

Snijders CJ, Slagter AH, Van Strik R, Vleeming A, Stoeckart R, Stam HJ. Why leg crossing? The influence of common postures on abdominal muscle activity. *Spine,* 1995; 20(18):1989-1993.

Vleeming A, Pool-Goudzwaard AL, Stoeckart R, van Wingerden JP, Snijders CJ. The posterior layer of the thoracolumbar fascia; its function in load transfer from spine to legs. *Spine,* 1995; 10(7):7353-758.

Chapter Nine

Inman VT, Ralston HJ, Todd F. *Human Walking.* Baltimore, Md: Williams and Wilkins; 1981.

Kapanji IA. *The Physiology of the Joints III: The Trunk and Vertebral Column.* 2nd ed. Edinburgh, Scotland: Churchill Livingstone; 1974.

Lee D. *The Pelvic Girdle: An Approach to the Examination and Treatment of the Lumbo-Pelvic-Hip Region,* New York, NY: Churchill Livingstone; 1999.

Panjabi MM. The stabilizing system of the spine. I: function, dysfunction, adaptation, and enhancement. *J Spinal Discord.* 1992; 5(4):383-389.

Sapsford RR, Hodges PW, Richardson CA. Activation of the abdominal muscles is a normal response to contraction of the pelvic floor. Presented at: the International Continence Society 27th Annual Meeting; September 23-26, 1997; Yokohama, Japan.

Vleeming A, Pool-Goudzwaard AL, Stoeckart R, van Wingerden JP, Snijders CJ. The posterior layer of the thoracolumbar fascia: its function in load transfer from spine to legs. *Spine.* 1995; 10(7):753-758.

Chapter Ten

Gershon H. *The Second Brain.* New York; Harper Collins, 1998.

Howard F. *Pelvic Pain: Diagnosis and Management.* New York: Lippincott Williams & Wilkins, 2000.

Hulme J. *Geriatric Incontinence: A Behavior and Exercise Approach to Treatment.* Missoula, Mont: Phoenix Publishing; 1999.

Inman VT, Ralston HJ, Todd F. *Human Walking.* Baltimore, Md: Williams and Wilkins; 1981.

Murray MD. Gait as a total pattern of movement. *Am J Phyl Med.* 1967; 46:290.

Scully R, Barnes M. *Physical Therapy.* New York, NY: Lippincott Co; 1989.

Travell J, Simons D: *Myofascial Pain & Dsyfunction The Trigger Point Manual.* Baltimore: Williams & Wilkins, 1983.

Wyke BD. Articular neurology and manipulative therapy. In: Glasgow EF, Twomyey LT, Scull ER, Kleynhans AM (ed) *Aspects of Manipulative Therapy.* 2nd ed. Melbourne, Australia: Churchill Livingstone; 1985:p72.

Chapter Eleven and Twelve

Howard F. *Pelvic Pain: Diagnosis and Management.* New York: Lippincott Williams & Wilkins, 2000.

Palter S ed. *Chronic Pelvic Pain. Infertility and Reproductive Medicine Clinics of North America.* Philadelphia: W.B. Saunders, 1999.

Rocker I ed. *Pelvic Pain in Women: Diagnosis and Management.* New York: Springer-Verlag, 1989.

Steege J, Metzger D, Levy B. *Chronic Pelvic Pain: An Integrated Approach.* Philadelphia: W.B. Saunders, 1998.

Chapter Thirteen

Berner F. *Urinary Incontinence and Voiding Dysfuntion in Sexual Abuse Survivors. Women & Childrens Outreach,* Colorado Gynecology & Continence Center.

Douglas A et.al. Sexual and physical abuse in women with functional or organic gastrointestinal problems. *Annals of Internal Medicine* 113:828-833, 1990.

Howard F. *Pelvic Pain Diagnosis & Management.* New York: Lippincott Williams & Wilkins, 2000.

Hulme, J. *Fibromyalgia: A Handbook for Self Care & Treatment.* Missoula, Mont: Phoenix Publishing, 2000.

Walker EA et.al. Medical psychiatric symptoms in women with childhood sexual abuse. *Psychom Med* 54:658-664, 1992.

Chapter Fifteen

Bremer HJ et. al. *Disturbances of Amino Acid Metabolism.* Baltimore: Urban & Schwarzenberg, 1981.

Bueler P. *Talking to Yourself.* San Francisco: HarperCollins, 1991.

Lieberman S, Bruning N. *The Real Vitamin & Mineral Book.* Garden City Park, NY: Avery Publishing, 1997.

Ornstein R, Sobel D. *Healthy Pleasures.* New York: Addison-Wesley Publishing, 1989.

Penner B. *Managing Fibromyalgia. A Six-Week Course on Self Care.* Missoula, MT: Phoenix Publishing, 1997.

Pert C. *Molecules of Emotion. The Science Behind Mind-Body Medicine.* New York: Simon & Schuster, 1997.

Slagle P. *The Way Up From Down.* New York: Random House, 1987.

Travell J, Simons D. *Myofascial Pain & Dsyfunction The Trigger Point Manual*. Baltimore: Williams & Wilkins, 1983.

Yao J. *Acutherapy Acupuncture T.E.N.S. and Acupressure*. Libertyville, IL: Acutherapy Postgraduate Seminars, 1984.

Chapter Sixteen
Barral J. *Urogenital Manipulation*. Seattle: Eastland Press, 1993.
Davis P. Aromatherapy. New York. Barnes and Noble, 1988.

Fabian P. *Myofascial Strategies Workshop*. Sacred Heart Medical Center. Spokane, Wa., March 15-17, 1991.

Fehmi L, Shor S. *Open Focus Workshop*. Helena, MT: Carroll College, June 8-10, 2201.

Fischer-Rizzi S. *Complete Aromatherapy Handbook: Essential Oils for Radiant Health*. NewYork: Sterling Publishing, 1990.

Galloway N. The Challenge of a Painful Bladder. In: Conner WH, ed. *Mediguide to Urology,* New York, NY: Lawrence DellaCarte Publishing, 1994.

Robbins J. *A Symphony in the Brain*. New York: Atlantic Monthly Press, 2000.

Sears B. *Enter the Zone*. New York: harper Collins Publishing, 1995.

Teitelbaum J. *From Fatigued to Fantastic A Manual for Moving Beyond Chronic Fatigue and Fibromyalgia*. Garden City Park, NY: Avery Publishing, 1996.

Tyler V. *Honest Herbal*. New York: Haworth Press, 1993.

Whitefield C. *Memory and Abuse*. Deerfield Beach, FL: Health Communications, Inc., 1995.

Order Form

Beyond Kegels: Fabulous Four (Book 1)   ____@$14.95 = $_____

Beyond Kegels: Personal Care Kit   ____@$39.00 = $_____

Geriatric Incontinence: A Behavioral &
Exercise approach to Treatment   ____@$29.95 = $_____

Beyond Kegels Book II: A Clinicians Guide ____@$85.95 = $_____

Physiological Quieting Tape   ____@$10.00 = $_____

Physiological Quieting CD   ____@$15.00 = $_____

Beyond Kegels Videotape   ____@$49.00 = $_____

Fibromyalgia: A Handbook for
Self Care & Treatment   ____@$14.95 = $_____

Pelvic Pain and Low Back Pain   ____@$24.95 = $_____

Subtotal $_____

Shipping/Handling $_____

SHIPPING/HANDLING

ORDER AMOUNT	GROUND
$00.01 – $18.00	$ 3.50
$18.01 – $35.00	$ 5.00
$35.01 – $50.00	$ 6.00
$50.01 – $75.00	$ 7.50
$75.01 – $100.00	$ 8.50
$100.01 – $150.00	$10.00

**Please Send Check/Credit Card
Money Order to:**
Phoenix Publishing
P.O. Box 8231, Missoula, MT 59807
1-800-549-8371
www.phoenixpub.com

TOTAL Cost of Order $_____

Name _____

Address _____

_____

City _____State _____Zip _____

Telephone (____) _____